Florida's Backyard

By

Carrie Hanna

ISBN: 0-7596-4801-8 (E-book)
ISBN: 0-7596-4802-6 (Paperback)
ISBN: 0-7596-4803-4 (RocketBook)
ISBN: 1-4033-8537-8 (Dustjacket)

This book is printed on acid free paper.

1stBooks - rev. 10/25/02

Table of Contents

Acknowledgements

Florida's Backyard is more a work of passion than a work of art. I have been fortunate to have the support of my family and numerous friends who encouraged me to convert my love of cooking and entertaining into a book. Naturally, I have many people to thank.

I would like to thank my family, especially my mom and dad who inspired me to begin cooking at a young age. Although my dad is not a "kitchen" man, both of my parents are barbecue aficionados and love the great outdoors. Mother is a true cook, the kind that never uses a recipe, only her senses.

I would also like to thank my stepsons, Paul, Josh and Carlton, who have never minded being my "guinea pigs" with my experimental meals. Thank you for wonderful memories of fun, family dinners. Paul's immense creativity was especially crucial to the editing and creative process and I truly enjoy sharing a love of cooking with him.

To my very dear friends and my sisters Joan and Cat, for their unending enthusiasm and encouragement. For my testing team members, both professional and novice, who gave me honest criticism: Thank you so very much.

To my husband who has loved, supported and believed in me every step of way: Thank you for your patience with this project and for having such a healthy appetite.

Finally, to my triplets, Cameron, Mark and Zan: Thank you for making every day a beautiful challenge.

Florida's Backyard

Introduction

I was always meant to write a cookbook. From the time I was a young girl, I would rummage through my mom's recipe drawer, which was filled with newspaper and magazine clippings and hand-written notes she had gathered from watching Julia Child or the Galloping Gourmet. It was a great way to pass the time and get ideas for new creations that I could make in the kitchen. My mom preferred cooking by trial and error and rarely used any of the hundreds of recipes tucked in her drawer. It was just "a little of this, a little of that." Dad often commented that her dishes never tasted the same way twice!

My parents are Miami natives and are among the few Floridians who still say, "My-a-mah." We grew up with all kinds of fresh produce in our backyard. Oranges, grapefruit, avocados, lemons and limes were perfect complements to the fresh fish my dad caught in his spare time. We spent summer vacations with friends in the Florida Keys and feasted on yellowtail snapper, lobster, hogfish, and conch all served with a side of hushpuppies and black beans and rice. I remember wandering through a neighbor's backyard and plucking fresh honeybell oranges from the trees, peeling away the thick rind, taking a bite and allowing the sweet juices to drip down my chin. So, it is only natural that *Florida's Backyard* would reflect the uncomplicated lifestyle of my childhood.

My mom's cooking style inspired me to experiment with my own recipes. I have always enjoyed trying new combinations, flavors and textures. Little did I know that all of this exploration would build into a passion for cooking and entertaining. I have been able to apply my first-hand knowledge to ideas that I have picked up from watching, testing and tasting the bounty of food from Florida and the Caribbean. And I have to say, what a delicious journey it has been!

It is both fortunate and exciting that Florida's cuisine and culinary resources have been the focus of the cooking world over the past several years. People across the country are learning to appreciate cooking with fresh, exotic fruits, as well as vegetables and a variety of seafood. Fresh fish has arrived on the scene with incredible popularity because of its increased availability across the country and its nutritional benefits. Renowned chefs have worked wonders bringing attention to the "Floribbean" and "New World" cuisine that originated in Florida and that both tourists and locals crave. *Florida's Backyard* captures the best of these techniques and dynamic flavors, but places them on a more manageable, less intimidating level.

The magic of *Florida's Backyard* is its relaxed approach to cooking and entertaining. For those of us with tight schedules, cooking should be easy so we don't lose interest and order out. Most of my recipes can be put together in less than an hour. The ingredients are found at most grocery stores and my cooking techniques are all within the scope of most home cooks. I have incorporated suggestions for variations and substitutions, and made recommendations of basic items to keep readily available. I have also included tips on buying and preparing fish. Basic equipment suggestions and ideas for stocking the pantry will keep you ready to create a meal on the spur of the moment.

Finally, I have included recommendations for entertaining, complete with a planning guide and checklist, menu ideas, party themes and tips for creating a memorable dining experience. *Florida's Backyard* was designed to be a cookbook that people use often. My hope is that this cookbook will give you some new favorite recipes and inspire you to create and have fun in your own kitchen.

To me, cooking for others is a gesture of love and caring that fills a home with an unparalleled character and warmth. It is also a creative outlet that satisfies and soothes the soul. I hope that *Florida's Backyard* will take you on an adventure with new flavors and culinary experiences. Whether you are a native Floridian, transplant or frequent visitor, may you discover a wealth of new ideas and insights that will help you to enjoy the bounty of our beautiful backyard!

Chapter 1

Starters and Salads

Abaco Conch Fritters with Two Sauces:
Pink Tartar Sauce
Apricot Horseradish Sauce
Triple-Cheese Shrimp Quesadillas
Avocado Bruschetta
Endive Spears with Goat Cheese and Pineapple
Lobster Cocktail with Mustard Sauce
Asparagus with Dilled Yogurt Horseradish Dip
Smoky Sweet Potato Soup
Carrot Ginger Soup
Chilled Roasted Pepper and Mango Soup
Avocado and Roasted Corn Soup
Summer Primavera Salad
Asparagus and Tomato Salad
Spinach Salad with Warm Strawberry Dressing
Wild Greens with Mango Vinaigrette
West End Conch Salad
Warm Hazelnut-Crusted Goat Cheese Salad with Raspberry Vinaigrette
Mixed Greens with Berries and Honey-Laced Citrus Vinaigrette
Spinach and Dried Fruit Salad with Lemon Vinaigrette
Summer Salad with Lemon Basil Ginger Vinaigrette

ABACO CONCH FRITTERS
WITH
TWO SAUCES

Island hopping through the Abacos in the Bahamas is my idea of a real vacation! No phones, no television, no newspapers—just a good book, reggae music and a nice breeze. My major accomplishment on my numerous Bahamas vacations over the years has been perfecting this recipe for conch fritters. These are as authentic as you can get, with tasty bites of sweet conch enveloped in a light, spicy batter.

4 medium conch, cleaned, skinned, pounded with a
     mallet and diced into ¼-inch to ½-inch cubes
½ green pepper, diced
1 small onion, diced
½ teaspoon garlic powder
2 eggs, beaten with ½ cup milk
1 and ¾-2 cups self-rising flour
1 Tablespoon hot sauce
Salt and pepper to taste
Hot oil for deep-frying (preferably peanut oil)

Combine conch, green pepper, onion and garlic powder in mixing bowl. Add egg mixture and stir to combine. Add flour a bit at a time until mixture resembles loose cookie dough (but not quite as stiff). Drop batter by Tablespoons into hot oil and deep fry until golden, about 4-5 minutes. Serve with Pink Tartar Sauce or Apricot Horseradish Sauce.

Makes 24-30 fritters.

Quick Tip: Place conch inside plastic bag before pounding with a mallet, to save yourself time during clean up!

PINK TARTAR SAUCE

This is my version of the traditional pink sauce that is served with fritters in the Florida Keys and throughout the Bahamas. It is also delicious with the fried fish of your choice.

½ medium onion, finely chopped
2 Tablespoons Heinz India relish or pickle relish
½ cup light or low-fat mayonnaise
¼ cup chili sauce
2 Tablespoons lemon juice
2 teaspoons hot sauce

Mix all ingredients together in a bowl. Mixture should be pink. Serve with conch fritters or fried fish.

Makes 1 and ½ cups.

APRICOT HORSERADISH SAUCE

A sweet and spicy dipping sauce for fritters or fish, this tangy condiment has a tasty "bite" to it that is unforgettable!

½ cup apricot preserves
2 Tablespoons honey
2 Tablespoons horseradish
1 Tablespoon lemon juice

Combine apricot preserves, honey, horseradish and lemon over low heat in small saucepan and stir until smooth. Cool and serve with conch fritters.
Makes ¾ cup.

TRIPLE-CHEESE SHRIMP QUESADILLAS

These popular, Mexican-inspired appetizers are surprisingly uncomplicated to make. I mastered the recipe and technique years ago. They are perfect for any party, although you would not want them falling out of a piñata! This version combines tender shrimp, crisp vegetables and a blending of cheeses for an inviting treat.

8 medium-size flour tortillas
½ pound medium or large fresh shrimp, shelled and deveined
2 teaspoons olive oil
1 clove garlic, minced
1 zucchini, julienned
½ pound mushrooms, sliced
1 cup fresh or frozen corn, cooked
1 red pepper, diced
1 jalapeno, seeded and minced
½ cup fresh cilantro, chopped (optional)
Salt and pepper to taste
4 ounces Monterey Jack cheese, shredded
4 ounces medium-to-sharp cheddar cheese, shredded
4 ounces goat cheese, crumbled

Accompaniments:
Sour cream
Salsa
Chopped avocado

Preheat oven to 350 degrees. In large, non-stick skillet, heat one teaspoon olive oil over medium-high heat. Season shrimp with salt and pepper and sauté in skillet until pink and firm, about 3 minutes per side. Remove from heat and let cool. Wipe skillet with paper towel and use it to heat one teaspoon of olive oil over medium-high heat. Sauté garlic until fragrant. Add zucchini, corn and jalapeno, and sauté until mixture begins to brown. Add mushrooms and peppers and continue to sauté until just tender, about 3-5 minutes. Season with salt and pepper to taste and season with fresh cilantro. Remove from skillet and set aside. Wipe same skillet, spray with non-stick spray and heat over medium-high heat. Place open tortillas in skillet one at a time. Add some shrimp, vegetable filling and cheeses to tortilla. Heat tortilla for 2-3 minutes until just crisp on outside. Use spatula to fold tortilla once, then heat another 2 minutes, until cheeses begin to melt. Repeat process for each tortilla.

If large, non-stick skillet is not available, use following method: Place tortillas on cookie sheets and lightly toast in oven about 5 minutes per side. When all tortillas have been toasted, assemble by placing four tortillas separately onto four large pieces of aluminum foil. Divide shrimp among tortillas, spread vegetable filling on shrimp and sprinkle three cheeses evenly over vegetable filling. Place second tortilla on top of cheese layer and wrap "sandwich" completely with foil. Place quesadillas in oven for another 8-10 minutes or until cheese melts. Remove from oven and cut each quesadilla into quarters or eighths. Serve on platter with sour cream and salsa.

Serves 6-8.

> *Quick Tip: Add some tropical flair to these quesadillas by using one of my fruit salsas as an accompaniment such as Avocado Salsa, Papaya Salsa, or Papaya-Yellow Tomato Salsa. For variations on the recipe, try different filling ingredients including diced pineapple, diced red onion or 1 cup rinsed and drained black beans. Sounds like a quesadilla party to me!*

AVOCADO BRUSCHETTA

The divine avocado is full of vitamins and has a flavor entirely its own. Here, avocado lends itself to the simple sophistication of a crisp, garlic bruschetta, creating an appetizer perfect for parties, cocktail hours or a light snack. You can also make an extra batch of avocado salsa and serve it with grilled shrimp.

1 avocado, cubed
2 plum tomatoes, seeded and diced
2 scallions, chopped
Juice of 1 lime
1 Tablespoon white wine vinegar
1 Tablespoon olive oil
2 teaspoons Tiger Sauce (or hot sauce of your choice)
½ teaspoon white pepper
½ teaspoon salt
½ teaspoon garlic powder
1 baguette fresh French or Italian bread, sliced diagonally
    in ½-inch slices
1 Tablespoon olive oil
1 clove garlic, minced
½ teaspoon coarse salt
¼ cup fresh cilantro, chopped

In medium bowl, combine first 10 ingredients and mix well. Let sit for minimum of 30 minutes (up to 2 hours), covered, in refrigerator. Preheat oven to 350 degrees. On cookie sheet, lay bread slices flat. In small bowl, using mortar and pestle, mash garlic, salt and olive oil. Brush olive oil mixture onto bread slices. Toast in oven for 8 minutes. Turn and toast another 4 minutes or until golden on both sides. Cool slightly. Top each bread slice with spoonful of avocado salsa and garnish with chopped fresh cilantro.

Makes 2 cups of salsa and 24 bruschetta.

ENDIVE SPEARS
WITH
GOAT CHEESE AND PINEAPPLE

Here is a simple but elegant appetizer that is perfect for a small dinner party or to dress up a buffet table. The contrasting flavors will lend a tasty and interesting introduction to any number of main courses. Placing the endive leaves on a circular plate and using a colorful centerpiece makes an impressive presentation. And, best of all, this recipe makes entertaining a breeze.

    24 Belgian endive leaves, rinsed and patted dry
    6 ounces goat cheese
    1 cup fresh pineapple, chopped in medium dice
    1 cup red seedless grapes, halved

Bring goat cheese to room temperature. Delicately spread about 1 Tablespoon of goat cheese into tips of endive leaves (toward core) and place 2-3 diced pineapple pieces at center, alternating with 2 grape halves. Place on circular plate, with pineapple pointing toward center. For centerpiece, use bowl of fresh strawberries or grapes, or assortment of olives.

Serves 6-8.

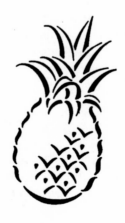

LOBSTER COCKTAIL
WITH
MUSTARD SAUCE

Any native will tell you that Florida Lobster is superior to its New England cousin. The spiny lobster, or crawfish as it is also known, is distinctive in its flavor and carries most of its edible meat in its tail. Every year during "Sportsman's Weekend," divers and snorkelers head for the coast to bag their limit of lobster. With any luck, a refrigerator full of tails is their reward. Here is my version of a shrimp cocktail, prepared with steamed lobster and a tangy mustard dipping sauce.

2 or 3 Florida lobster tails (small-to-medium)
½ cup mayonnaise
½ cup sour cream
¼ cup Dijon mustard
2 teaspoons Worcestershire sauce
2 teaspoons hot sauce
Juice of one lemon
1 Tablespoon fresh parsley, chopped
Dash of white pepper (to taste)

Place lobster tails in large pot and add about 2 inches of water. Cover and place over high heat. Steam tails for 7-10 minutes, then cool. Split tails and peel meat away from shell. Chill in refrigerator for 1 hour to 1 day in advance. In medium bowl, combine next 7 ingredients and stir until smooth. Season with pepper. Cut lobster into 1- or 2-inch pieces and serve on platter with mustard sauce for dipping.

Serves 6.

> *Quick Tip: You can cut calories and fat in this dish by substituting low-fat mayonnaise and reduced-fat sour cream. It's equally tasty both ways.*

ASPARAGUS
WITH
DILLED YOGURT HORSERADISH DIP

For all asparagus lovers, here is a refreshing and elegant appetizer that is also quick and easy to prepare. Although the true season for asparagus is mid-March through June, imported asparagus can often be found during other months of the year. This creamy yogurt dip has a pleasant bite that adds a spark to brightly blanched asparagus or any crunchy crudite.

½ cup plain non-fat yogurt
¼ cup regular or reduced-fat sour cream
1½ Tablespoons horseradish
1 teaspoon honey mustard
1 Tablespoon coarse grain Dijon mustard
2 teaspoons fresh dill
½ teaspoon lemon zest
1 pound asparagus, trimmed and blanched

In medium bowl, combine first 8 ingredients. Chill 30 minutes to 1 hour and serve with blanched asparagus. You can also serve this dip with carrots, pea pods, blanched broccoli florets and cherry tomatoes.

Serves 4-6.

> *Quick Tip: What is lemon zest? Lemon zest is the outermost portion of the lemon rind, which contains oils that enhance the flavor of a dish. Use a zester, which can be purchased at any kitchen store, to peel this portion of the rind. You can also use a very sharp vegetable peeler to remove only the colorful outer portion of the skin.*

SMOKY SWEET POTATO SOUP

Sweet potatoes just have to be one of world's most perfect foods! Dense with flavor and full of vitamins A and C and potassium, they lend themselves to a variety of recipes. Typically a Southern favorite, they are also popular in the rest of the country and often used in Latin American cooking as well. Here is a sensational soup full of diverse characteristics that blend to make a memorable first course.

> 2 Tablespoons butter
> 1½ pounds sweet potatoes, peeled and sliced into ¼-inch rounds
> 1 large onion, diced (yellow or Vidalia)
> 2 (14-ounce) cans vegetable broth
> 1 cup water
> 1 cinnamon stick
> 1 medium ham hock (about 10 ounces)
> ½ teaspoon nutmeg
> ½-1 teaspoon white pepper
> ½ teaspoon liquid smoke (optional)
> 1 cup whole milk
> 1 Granny Smith apple, peeled, cored and sliced into ¼-inch slices

In large saucepan, melt butter over medium heat and add onions. Sauté onions until softened, about 5 minutes. Add potatoes, cinnamon stick, vegetable broth and ham hock. Cover and bring to simmer. Uncover and continue to simmer until potatoes and ham hock are tender, 20-25 minutes. Remove from heat and cool slightly. Remove ham hock and cinnamon stick and puree soup in batches. Return mixture to pan over low heat. Add pepper, nutmeg and liquid smoke and stir to combine thoroughly. Add milk in a slow stream and stir well. Garnish with sliced Granny Smith apples.

Serves 6.

CARROT GINGER SOUP

Carrots and ginger create a bright and enticing partnership abundant with flavor. Full of beta-carotene, the parent to Vitamin A, carrots make an unrivalled addition to any menu. This sensational, refreshing soup will help you to appreciate carrots in a whole new and natural way.

2 Tablespoons butter
1 medium onion, chopped
2 Tablespoons fresh ginger, chopped
2 Tablespoons brown sugar
3 cups carrots, chopped, or baby carrots
4 cups vegetable broth
1 cup water
½ cup half-and-half or whole milk
Salt and pepper to taste
Fresh mint sprigs
Sour cream for garnish.

In large pot, melt butter over medium heat, add onion and ginger and sauté until onion is translucent. Add carrots, vegetable broth and water and simmer until carrots are tender, about 25 minutes. Cool slightly. Puree soup mixture in batches and return to pan over low heat. Add salt and pepper to taste and pour milk in stream, stirring well to combine. Serve with dollop of sour cream and mint sprig.

Serves 8-10.

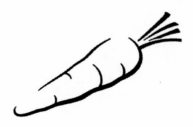

11

CHILLED ROASTED PEPPER
AND
MANGO SOUP

Refreshing and cool is what this soup is all about. This blend of extraordinary ingredients will definitely both whet and satisfy your appetite!

3 yellow peppers, halved
½ cup vegetable broth
2 medium mangoes, peeled and sliced
1 cup mango nectar*
Juice of 1 large lime
1 Tablespoon fresh ginger, minced
2 teaspoons hot sauce
2 Tablespoons rice vinegar
Dash of cayenne pepper
Sour cream for garnish
3 Tablespoons fresh mint, chopped

*Available in juice section at most major grocery stores.

Prepare grill. Place peppers on hot grill skin side down, and cook about 5 minutes per side or until slightly charred. Place in plastic zipper bag, paper bag or bowl covered with plastic wrap, and steam for 15 minutes. Skin with paring knife and slice into quarters. (Alternately, prepare broiler and broil peppers skin side up for about 5 minutes per side or until slightly charred. Place in plastic zipper bag, paper bag or bowl and steam for 15 minutes.)

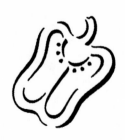

In blender or food processor, puree yellow peppers, add vegetable broth and puree until smooth. Add mangoes and puree until smooth. Add mango nectar, lime juice, ginger, hot sauce, rice vinegar and cayenne pepper and blend well. You can puree in batches. Strain through sieve into large bowl, pressing pulp and solids to extract all liquid. Discard pulp. Cover and chill soup 1-2 hours. Serve with dollop of sour cream and garnish with mint.

Serves 4.

Quick Tip: To peel and slice mangoes, use a sharp knife, starting at wide end of fruit and peeling in a circle until you reach the opposite end, then slice mango parallel to pit, experimenting until you find direction of pit. You should be able to slice the 2 large halves from their side of the pit, then 2 smaller halves from sides running against the pit. Proceed with chopping mango as directed in recipe.

AVOCADO AND ROASTED CORN SOUP

Florida avocados have one-half less fat and one-third fewer calories than California avocados. But my Aunt Carol, who grows avocados in southern Spain, believes hers are best. My family's ongoing "avocado competition" inspired me to create this sensational soup!

2 ears fresh corn, husked
1 Tablespoon butter, melted
1 large Florida avocado, peeled and coarsely chopped
1 Tablespoon olive oil
1 jalapeno, seeded and chopped
2 cloves garlic, minced
½ medium Vidalia onion, chopped
2 cups canned vegetable broth
½ cup milk
¼ cup fresh lime juice
1 teaspoon hot sauce, preferably Tiger Sauce
1 teaspoon cumin
1/3 cup pumpkin seeds, toasted and salted
¼ cup fresh cilantro, chopped
Salt and pepper to taste

Prepare grill. Place corn over medium-high heat and coat with butter. Grill until golden brown, about 10 minutes. Remove and cool to room temperature. Carve kernels from cob and set aside. In medium, non-stick skillet, heat olive oil over medium-high heat and sauté garlic, onion and jalapeno until soft and translucent, about 5 minutes. In blender, puree three-quarters of chopped avocado with jalapeno, garlic and onion mixture and one-half of vegetable broth. Add milk and blend. Add lime juice, cumin and hot sauce and blend. Add remaining vegetable broth and puree until smooth. Season with salt and pepper to taste. Chill for one hour. Stir in roasted corn and remaining avocado chunks. Garnish with pumpkin seeds and pinch of cilantro.

Serves 4.

> *Quick Tip: It's okay to substitute 1 cup frozen corn kernels, thawed, for fresh corn. Toast in skillet over medium-high heat with 1 teaspoon olive oil until just golden brown.*

SUMMER PRIMAVERA SALAD

One of the essential elements of summer is a killer pasta salad. For picnics, parties, beach, boat or lake, this salad will become a mainstay. You'll find yourself making it all year long, just to bring back nostalgic memories of easy summer days and laid-back barbecues.

For vinaigrette:
> 6 Tablespoons olive oil
> 3 Tablespoons balsamic vinegar
> 2 teaspoons Dijon mustard
> 1 Tablespoon lemon juice
> ½ teaspoon garlic powder to taste

For salad:
> 1 pound fusilli pasta, cooked and cooled to room temperature
> 1 red pepper, diced
> ½ basket cherry tomatoes (about 10), halved
> 1 carrot, julienned
> 1/3 red onion, diced
> 10 green olives, sliced
> 10 calamata olives, sliced
> ½ cup crumbled feta cheese
> ½ cup fresh basil, chopped

Whisk together vinegar, mustard, lemon juice and garlic powder. Add olive oil and whisk until emulsified. Combine next 7 ingredients in bowl and toss with dressing until well blended. Add feta cheese and basil and toss again. Chill and serve.

Serves 6-8 as side dish.

ASPARAGUS AND TOMATO SALAD

There is no replacement for the vibrant flavor and character of good, vine-ripened tomatoes, and Florida produces more tomatoes than any other state in the country. I created this simple salad in celebration of our best crop, which peaks during the summer. The delicious blend of asparagus, blue cheese and basil provides the perfect complement for ripe, juicy tomatoes.

2 fresh, vine-ripened tomatoes, sliced
1 bunch asparagus, blanched
3 Tablespoons fresh basil, chopped
2 ounces Danish blue cheese, crumbled
2 Tablespoons balsamic vinegar
½ teaspoon kosher salt
2 Tablespoons extra-virgin olive oil
Fresh ground pepper to taste

Place sliced tomatoes and asparagus on platter. Sprinkle with blue cheese, basil and kosher salt. Drizzle with balsamic vinegar and olive oil. Chill for 30 minutes. Season with pepper to taste.

Serves 4-6.

> *Quick Tip: Tomatoes were meant to be served at room temperature. Refrigeration will cause them to lose their flavor and texture. Always store tomatoes at room temperature, on a windowsill away from direct light, on a tray or in a bowl. Remember, when placed in a decorative bowl, tomatoes make a beautiful centerpiece!*

SPINACH SALAD
WITH
WARM STRAWBERRY DRESSING

Spinach salad is traditionally dressed with a warm dressing, but you've never had one quite like this. Low in fat and high in flavor, this fusion of balsamic vinegar, strawberries and maple syrup offers a tangy contrast to the buttery flavor of blue cheese.

2 cups fresh spinach leaves, cleaned and spun dry
2 cups romaine lettuce, torn into pieces
1 yellow pepper, julienned
1 cup fresh strawberries, sliced
2 shallots, coarsely chopped
1/3 cup plus 1 Tablespoon balsamic vinegar
2 Tablespoons strawberry preserves
1 Tablespoon pure maple syrup
3 Tablespoons fresh orange juice
2 Tablespoons olive oil
1 Tablespoon walnut oil
¼ cup toasted walnuts
4 ounces blue cheese, crumbled
Fresh sliced mushrooms, if desired

In skillet sprayed with cooking spray, heat shallots over medium-low heat and sauté until they begin to turn brown. Add 1/3 cup balsamic vinegar and simmer shallots until balsamic is reduced by half, about 10 minutes. Add ½ cup strawberries and sauté until just soft, 3-4 minutes. Add preserves and maple syrup and stir until dissolved in mixture. Set mixture aside and let cool, slightly. Meanwhile, combine remaining spinach, yellow pepper, strawberries and mushrooms (if desired). Transfer shallot, vinegar and strawberry mixture to blender. Add orange juice, olive oil and walnut oil and puree until smooth. Return mixture to skillet, over low heat, and heat until just warm. Toss salad with warm dressing, sprinkle on toasted walnuts and blue cheese and toss once more.

Serves 4-6.

WILD GREENS
WITH
MANGO VINAIGRETTE

I don't like boring salads, and this combination of ingredients is anything but! It brings together the luscious fruit flavors of mangoes and berries, and tosses them with the subtle sophistication of buttery blue cheese. It's truly addictive.

For salad:
      4 cups mixed baby greens
      6-8 mushrooms, washed and sliced
      1 yellow pepper, julienned
      ¾ pint fresh strawberries, sliced
      4 ounces blue cheese
      ½ cup walnuts, toasted and coarsely chopped

For vinaigrette: (makes ¾ cup)
      3 Tablespoons mango vinegar*
      ½ cup mango nectar
      1 Tablespoon olive oil
      1 Tablespoon walnut oil
      3 teaspoons Dijon mustard
      ¼ cup fresh basil, chopped
      1 Tablespoon lemon juice
      1 shallot, finely chopped
      1 Tablespoon fresh ginger, finely minced

*Available at gourmet markets and Williams-Sonoma.

In large bowl, combine lettuces, mushrooms, peppers and strawberries. In medium bowl, combine vinegar, nectar, mustard, shallots, basil, lemon juice and ginger, and whisk until smooth. Whisk in oils until emulsified. Toss salad with dressing, using only enough to coat lettuce lightly. Add walnuts and blue cheese and toss again. Serve onto salad plates.

Serves 4-6.

WEST END CONCH SALAD

West End on Grand Bahamas Island is a simple, uncomplicated treasure. Just two hours from the Palm Beach County coast (by way of most power boats), the area abounds with fish, lobster and conch. Similar to ceviche, conch salad is a native island staple. Marinating it briefly in lime juice adds flavor and tenderizes the sweet morsels. Serve it as an appetizer with crackers, or on its own for a lazy afternoon lunch. There is no wrong way to eat conch salad—just ask any Bahamas native!

4 conch, cleaned, with skin removed
1 small Vidalia onion, chopped
1 red pepper, chopped
½ yellow pepper, chopped
1 jalapeno pepper, seeded and chopped
1 large tomato, seeded and chopped
½ cup fresh lime juice
1 teaspoon hot sauce
2 Tablespoons fresh cilantro, chopped
Salt and pepper to taste

Dice conch and combine with vegetables. Add lime juice and hot sauce and stir to combine. Add cilantro, season with salt and pepper and chill for 1 hour minimum before serving.

Serves 6-8.

> *Quick Tip: Most conch sold in the United States is already frozen. Unlike most shellfish, however, it freezes well and maintains its flavor. Seafood markets usually sell it already cleaned, but ask to be sure.*

WARM HAZELNUT-CRUSTED GOAT CHEESE SALAD
WITH
RASPBERRY VINAIGRETTE

Tangy goat cheese, sweet raspberries and luxurious hazelnuts make a salad that's a must for entertaining. The presentation and flavors will impress even the most discriminating of guests. This dish is deceivingly simple to create, so don't restrict it to special occasions; indulge yourself anytime!

For salad:
>   8 ounces mixed baby greens
>   ½ yellow pepper, julienned
>   1 ripe Anjou pear, cored and sliced lengthwise
>   6 ounces goat cheese
>   1 egg white
>   ½ cup hazelnuts, toasted and finely ground
>   1/3 cup dried cranberries

For vinaigrette:
>   ¼ cup raspberry vinegar
>   2 Tablespoons raspberry jam or seedless preserves
>   1 Tablespoon maple syrup
>   1 Tablespoon honey mustard
>   1 Tablespoon lemon juice
>   2 Tablespoons walnut oil
>   2 Tablespoons olive oil
>   2 Tablespoons fresh tarragon, chopped
>   Pinch of white pepper to taste

Place mixed baby greens and yellow peppers in bowl. Set aside. Preheat oven to 350 degrees. Spray cookie sheet with non-stick spray. Place egg white in small bowl with 1 Tablespoon of water and whisk to light foam. Slice goat cheese into 6 pieces, ½-inch wide. Dip into egg white and roll in toasted hazelnuts, coating evenly. Place on cookie sheet. Bake for 10 minutes; keep warm. In medium bowl, whisk raspberry vinegar, maple syrup, raspberry preserves, lemon juice and honey mustard until blended. Add walnut oil and olive oil and whisk until emulsified. Add tarragon, season lightly with pepper and whisk again. Add pears to salad mixture. Toss mixed greens with raspberry vinaigrette, using only a little to coat leaves. Place on plates; top with cheese disc and 1 Tablespoon cranberries.

Serves 4-6.

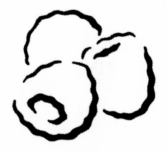

MIXED GREENS AND BERRIES
WITH
HONEY-LACED CITRUS VINAIGRETTE

This is the ultimate salad to serve when berries are at their freshest. Florida is known for its winter strawberry season, which starts in December and lasts through late spring. Here, I've tossed these sweet gems with honey-laced citrus vinaigrette and crisp greens, creating a cool and invigorating salad.

For vinaigrette:
   2 Tablespoons honey
   3 Tablespoons rice vinegar
   1 Tablespoon lemon juice
   1 teaspoon lemon zest
   ¼ cup fresh orange juice
   1 teaspoon orange zest
   2 teaspoons Dijon mustard
   2 Tablespoons olive oil
   Fresh cracked pepper to taste

For salad:
   4 cups mixed baby greens
   ½ cup fresh strawberries, sliced
   ¼ cup raspberries
   4 ounces goat cheese, crumbled
   ¼ cup sunflower seeds, toasted and salted
   2 Tablespoons dried cranberries

In small bowl, whisk together honey, vinegar, juices and mustard. Add orange and lemon zest, olive oil and fresh cracked pepper and whisk again until emulsified. In large bowl, toss baby greens with just enough dressing to coat. Add strawberries and raspberries and toss again, adding more dressing if necessary. Serve onto plates and sprinkle with crumbled goat cheese, dried berries and sunflower seeds. To store dressing, strain through sieve and put into air-tight container.

Serves 4.

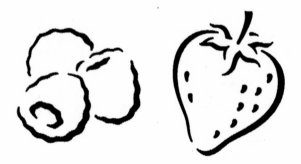

SPINACH AND DRIED FRUIT SALAD
WITH
LEMON VINAIGRETTE

This colorful spinach salad is loaded with wholesome ingredients. Tossed with sweet and sour vinaigrette, it's light and delicious and the perfect complement to fresh seafood.

For vinaigrette:
    3 Tablespoons red wine vinegar
    2 Tablespoons lemon juice
    1 Tablespoon lemon rind, freshly grated
    1 teaspoon sugar
    3 Tablespoons Dijon mustard
    3-4 Tablespoons olive oil

For salad:
    1 (12-ounce) package fresh spinach, cleaned, stemmed
       and coarsely chopped
    ¼ medium red onion, thinly sliced
    ¼ cup golden raisins
    ¼ cup dried cranberries
    ¼ cup dried apricots, chopped
    ½ cup dried figs, chopped
    2 Tablespoons sunflower seeds, toasted, salted

In medium bowl, combine vinegar, lemon juice, lemon rind, sugar and Dijon mustard and whisk until blended. Add the olive oil and whisk until emulsified. Set aside. In large bowl, combine chopped fresh spinach, onion and dried fruit. Toss with dressing until well blended. Sprinkle with sunflower seeds and serve onto plates.

Serves 4-6.

Variations:

- *Add feta or goat cheese for a more substantial salad.*
- *Try dried cherries or other dried berries, if available.*
- *If a called-for dried fruit is not available, double the amount of another fruit.*
- *Top with pan-seared shrimp for a main course salad*

SUMMER SALAD
WITH
LEMON BASIL GINGER VINAIGRETTE

There is something so summer-like about adding fruit to a green salad. If you are like I am, you keep a fresh bowl of fruit on your counter all year long. From May to September, when nectarines and plums are at their peak, this salad is just the "cooling-off" cure for hot summer days. This crisp, refreshing and colorful salad also adds an impressive display to picnics and outdoor parties.

For salad:
> 8 cups mixed baby greens
> 4 ounces feta cheese
> 1 medium plum, sliced
> 1 medium nectarine, sliced
> 6 fresh button mushrooms, sliced
> ½ yellow bell pepper, julienned

For dressing:
> 1/3 cup fresh lemon juice
> 3 Tablespoons white wine vinegar
> 6 Tablespoons olive oil
> 1/3 cup fresh basil
> 2 Tablespoons freshly grated ginger
> ½ teaspoon salt
> Dash of fresh ground pepper

In large bowl, mix salad ingredients together and toss lightly. In blender, combine lemon juice, vinegar, olive oil, fresh basil and ginger. Blend on medium until well blended. Add salt and pepper and blend again. Add dressing a little at a time, tossing until lettuce is barely coated. Store leftover dressing in refrigerator. It will keep 2-3 days.

Serves 4-6.

Chapter 2

Sidekicks

Crispy Jalapeno Olive Potatoes
Soulful Succotash
Sun-kissed Couscous
Roasted Yukon Gold Potatoes and Leeks
Island Rice
Coconut Curry Jasmine Rice

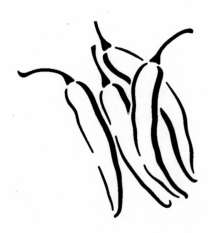

CRISPY JALAPENO OLIVE POTATOES

The jalapenos in this dish give a swift, spicy kick to simple, pan-seared potatoes. Crispy on the outside and tender on the inside, these potatoes are great with steak, fish or chicken.

> 2 pounds red potatoes, cleaned and cut into 2-inch wedges.
> 1 Tablespoon olive oil
> 8-10 jalapeno-stuffed olives
> 4 scallions, sliced
> 1 teaspoon Tiger Sauce or hot sauce of your choice

Place potatoes in large pot and cover with water. Bring to boil and cook for 15 minutes, until potatoes are just tender, but still firm when tested with a fork. Drain potatoes in colander. In large, non-stick skillet, heat olive oil over medium-high heat until hot but not smoking. Add potatoes and sauté about 5 minutes, stirring often until slightly tender. Add scallions, jalapeno-stuffed olives and Tiger Sauce, and stir until heated through. Cover and cook for 5 minutes until potatoes develop a golden-brown crust.

Serves 4—6.

> *Quick Tip: If you can't find jalapeno-stuffed olives, substitute 8-10 colossal green pimento-stuffed olives and 1 seeded, finely chopped jalapeno.*

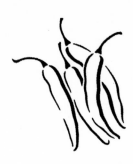

SOULFUL SUCCOTASH

Succotash is a traditional vegetable and bean dish originating in the Deep South. This updated version combines color, flavor and texture with wonderful Latin influences of black beans and spicy peppers. This also makes an excellent cold salad, so keep any leftovers!

1 Tablespoon olive oil
¼ teaspoon red pepper flakes
½ teaspoon cumin
½ teaspoon chili powder
2 cups fresh or frozen, thawed and drained corn kernels, cooked
1 red bell pepper, seeded and chopped
1 jalapeno pepper, seeded and finely chopped
1 cup canned black beans, drained and rinsed
3 scallions, sliced on diagonal into ½-inch pieces
1 Tablespoon fresh lime juice
1 Tablespoon hot sauce
¼ cup fresh cilantro, chopped
2 Tablespoons fresh chives, chopped

In non-stick skillet, heat olive oil and red pepper flakes over medium-high heat. Add corn kernels and sauté until barely golden, 2-3 minutes. Reduce heat to medium-low, add cumin and chili powder and stir to blend. Add red bell pepper and jalapeno pepper and sauté until red bell pepper is just tender, about 4 minutes. Add black beans, scallions, lime juice, hot sauce and cilantro and stir until heated through. Garnish with chives and serve as side dish.

Serves 6.

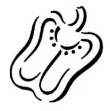

Sun-kissed Couscous

Couscous is one of my all-time favorite side dishes. It is easy and elegant, and you can toss it with a variety of ingredients. This combination is sensational, full of diverse flavors and textures. The fragrant blend of ginger, apricots and herbs, along with crunchy peppers and pine nuts, creates an impressive accompaniment for fish or chicken.

> 2 teaspoons olive oil
> ½ red bell pepper, chopped
> 4 scallions, sliced
> 1 Tablespoon fresh ginger, minced
> 1/3 cup dried apricots, chopped
> ¼ cup pine nuts, toasted
> ¼ cup fresh basil, chopped
> ¼ cup fresh mint, chopped
> 1 1/3 cup couscous
> 2 cups water
> ½ teaspoon fresh ground pepper
> Salt to taste

Heat olive oil in non-stick skillet over medium heat. Add red bell pepper, scallions and ginger, and sauté until vegetables are just tender. Add apricots and toss until heated through. Set mixture aside. In medium saucepan, heat water until boiling and add couscous. Cover and remove from heat. Let couscous stand for 5 minutes or until all water is absorbed. Fluff couscous with fork. Stir in red bell pepper mixture and add pine nuts, basil and mint. Combine well. Stir in pepper and season with salt to taste.

Makes 4-6 servings.

ROASTED YUKON GOLD POTATOES AND LEEKS

Yukon Gold potatoes have a buttery color and lush flavor that is enhanced by roasting. Here, they are blended with leeks, rosemary and thyme, all classic herbs for potatoes. Serve this dish with your favorite steak, chicken, lamb or pork entree.

1 pound Yukon Gold potatoes, cleaned and cut into quarters
2 leeks, sliced thin (retain only white and pale green parts)
1 Tablespoon fresh rosemary, chopped
1 Tablespoon fresh thyme, chopped
1 Tablespoon olive oil
1 garlic clove, minced
1 teaspoon coarse salt
Fresh cracked pepper

Preheat oven to 400 degrees. In large bowl, combine potatoes and leeks. In small bowl, combine olive oil and garlic. Drizzle olive oil and garlic mixture over potatoes and toss to coat. Add fresh herbs, salt and pepper and toss again. Spray shallow, 9-inch baking pan with non-stick spray. Put potato mixture into pan and roast until potatoes are tender and golden brown (about 35 minutes), stirring every 10-12 minutes to re-coat with herbs.

Serves 6.

ISLAND RICE

Inspired by the Bahamian tradition of combining peas and rice (there is actually a Bahamian Soca song named "Peas and Rice"), I have adapted my own, healthier version. Brown rice has a great texture, and can be paired with any extra. The addition of pecans and green peas boosts the naturally sweet and nutty flavors of this wholesome grain.

> 1 Tablespoon butter
> 1/3 cup yellow onion, finely chopped
> 1 cup brown rice
> 2 ¼ cups water
> 1 (10-ounce) package frozen green peas without sauce, thawed
> ½ cup pecans, toasted and coarsely chopped
> Salt and pepper to taste

In medium saucepan, heat 1 Tablespoon butter until melted. Add onion and sauté until translucent, about 3 minutes. Add rice and sauté 2 minutes. Add water and bring to boil. Cover and reduce heat, simmering until all water is absorbed, about 45-50 minutes. Add peas and pecans, season with salt and pepper and serve.

Serves 4—6.

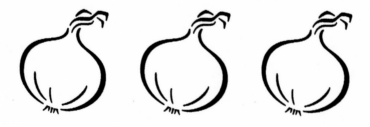

COCONUT CURRY JASMINE RICE

The mildly tropical flavors in this dish are sensational! A touch of spice and hint of coconut will make you feel as though you have been transported to a Caribbean island. Create your own innovative tropical menu or dress up any basic main course with this exotic accompaniment.

1½ Tablespoons butter
1 small onion, chopped
2 teaspoons curry powder
1/3 cup golden raisins
1 cup jasmine rice
1 cup light coconut milk*
½ cup vegetable broth or reduced-sodium vegetable broth
½ cup water
½ teaspoon salt
1 bay leaf

*If you can't find light coconut milk, use ½ cup regular coconut milk diluted with ½ cup water.

In heavy saucepan, melt butter and sauté onion until translucent. Add curry powder and rice and cook mixture 2 minutes, stirring constantly. Add raisins and continue stirring. Add coconut milk, broth, water, salt and bay leaf. Bring mixture to boil, cover and reduce to low simmer for about 20 minutes or until all liquid is absorbed. Add more water as needed, a little at a time, to keep rice from sticking. Remove bay leaf and season with additional salt and pepper if desired.

Serves 4-6.

Chapter 3

From the Sea

Grilled Native Snapper with Warm Black Bean Citrus Salsa
Herb-Crusted Yellowtail with Banana Ginger Salsa
Banana Ginger Salsa
Native Snapper with Banana Citrus Sauce
Crispy Yellowtail Parmesan
Spice-Rubbed Yellowtail with Nectarine Salsa
Native Snapper with Fresh Tomato, Olive and Caper Sauce
Grilled Mahi-Mahi with Stir-Fry Vegetables
Grilled Cobia with Papaya Salsa
Grilled Tuna with Puttanesca Relish
Stir-Fry Marinated Cobia
Herb-Sealed Grouper on the Grill
Roasted Red Pepper Shrimp and Black Bean Barbecue
Lemon Dill Shrimp Sauté
Tropical Shrimp Risotto
Pan-Seared Colossal Shrimp with Cranberry Orange Salsa
Cornmeal-Crusted Shrimp with Jalapeno Jelly
Shrimp Pasta with Mushrooms and Sun-dried Tomatoes
Dad's Best Broiled Lobster Tails with Herb Butter
Beer-Battered Bahamian Crawfish
Sweet Peppered Scallops
Pan-Seared Scallops with Papaya Yellow Tomato Salsa
Pan-Seared Scallops with Citrus Reduction
Skinny Crab and Asparagus Quiche

GRILLED NATIVE SNAPPER WITH WARM BLACK BEAN CITRUS SALSA

Considering that the main ingredients in this dish are native to the Florida Peninsula, this could be the state's signature recipe. Rich, citrus flavors such as oranges and lime blend beautifully with mild and flaky snapper. Hearty black beans, spicy peppers and the accompanying salsa make a wonderfully interesting combination.

¾-1 pound snapper filets

Marinade:
    ½ cup orange juice
    Juice of 1 lime
    1 Tablespoon honey mustard
    1 shallot, finely chopped
    ½ cup cilantro
    ½ cup basil
    1 garlic clove, minced

Salsa:
    2 teaspoons olive oil
    1 (15-ounce) can black beans, rinsed and drained
    1 navel orange, peeled, sectioned and coarsely chopped
    1 medium red pepper, coarsely chopped
    1/3 cup cilantro, chopped
    1 jalapeno, seeded and minced
    ¼ cup red wine vinegar
    1 garlic clove, minced
    1 shallot, minced

Mix first 7 ingredients and let fish marinate for at least 1 hour. Heat oil in non-stick skillet over medium-high heat. Sauté garlic, shallot and jalapeno until soft and fragrant, about 3 minutes. Add red peppers and cilantro and vinegar and reduce for 5-7 minutes. Add black beans and oranges and stir until heated through. Grill fish about 4 minutes per side, until cooked through. Spoon salsa on plate, place grilled fish on top and garnish with cilantro.

Serves 4.

HERB-CRUSTED YELLOWTAIL
WITH
BANANA GINGER SALSA

Because fresh herbs bring out so many enticing flavors, they make a delicious crust for most fish. I came up with this recipe after a weekend of fishing filled our refrigerator with yellowtail snapper. The golden herb coating, delicate flavor of the fish and fruity salsa combine to create a remarkable taste sensation.

1½ pounds yellowtail (approximately 4 medium filets)
    cleaned, skinned and trimmed
2/3 cup all-purpose flour
½ teaspoon salt
½ teaspoon black pepper
2/3 cup bread crumbs (homemade or commercial)
3 scallions, finely minced
½ cup fresh cilantro, finely minced
¼ cup fresh mint, finely minced
¼ teaspoon ground ginger
¼ teaspoon white pepper
¼ teaspoon salt
1 egg white, lightly beaten with 1 Tablespoon of water
2 Tablespoons olive oil

Dredge fish filets in flour seasoned with 1/4 teaspoon salt and 1/2 teaspoon black pepper. In shallow bowl or food processor, mix bread crumbs, scallions, cilantro, mint, ginger, 1/4 teaspoon salt and white pepper. Dip fish filets in egg white and coat with breadcrumb mixture. Refrigerate filets for 20 minutes. Heat olive oil in skillet over medium-high heat. Sauté filets 4-5 minutes per side or until crust is golden brown. Serve with Banana Ginger Salsa.

Serves 4.

Quick Tip: Making homemade breadcrumbs is easier than you think, and worth the nominal effort. Keep a stock of leftover baguettes or Italian loaves in your freezer. When you are ready to make breadcrumbs, thaw desired amount of bread and process to desired consistency in food processor.

BANANA GINGER SALSA

This has to be one of best fruit salsas you will ever try! Its uses are unending, its flavors unparalleled. Try this salsa with fish, shrimp, chicken or scallops, and it will surely become a favorite in your repertoire.

    1 just-ripe banana
    Juice of 1 lime
    1 Tablespoon brown sugar
    1 small-to-medium red pepper, coarsely chopped
    1 jalapeno, seeded and minced
    1 Tablespoon fresh ginger, minced
    3 scallions, sliced
    ¼ cup fresh cilantro, chopped
    1 Tablespoon fresh mint, chopped

Combine ingredients and let sit for 30 minutes before serving.

Makes 1¼ cups.

> *Quick Tip: Add some variation to this recipe with mild tropical fruits such as kiwi or papaya. They will add color and blend well with the other flavors.*

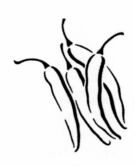

NATIVE SNAPPER WITH BANANA CITRUS SAUCE

From May until October, our house could be called "Florida Snapper Central," because we catch a variety of snapper nearly every weekend. Mutton, yellowtail, mangrove and lane are the most common varieties. They are all delicious, with a white flaky texture and mild flavor. A good fishmonger will offer a couple of varieties of snapper, including deep-water reds, mutton or yellowtail. This recipe showcases this wonderfully delicate fish, enhanced with gentle infusions of bananas, orange and ginger.

4 Florida snapper filets (about 1 ½ pounds)
½ cup flour
1 teaspoon paprika
Salt and pepper to taste
1 Tablespoon olive oil
¼ cup fresh-squeezed orange juice
1 Tablespoon white wine or sherry
1 Tablespoon fresh ginger, grated
2 Tablespoons lemon juice
2 Tablespoons brown sugar
2 bananas, quartered lengthwise
¼ cup macadamia nuts, toasted and chopped

Combine flour, paprika, salt and pepper. Dredge snapper filets in flour mixture to coat. Heat olive oil in non-stick skillet over medium-high heat. Sauté filets until golden brown, 2-3 minutes per side. Remove from pan, transfer to plate and keep warm. Reduce heat to medium. Add fresh orange juice to skillet along with wine, sherry, ginger, lemon, and brown sugar. Stir mixture and add bananas. Bring mixture to simmer and cook for 2 minutes. Pour sauce over filets and sprinkle with macadamia nuts.

Serves 4.

Quick Tip: To toast macadamia nuts, preheat oven to 325 degrees. Place nuts on cookie sheet and bake until just lightly browned and fragrant, about 15 minutes. Cool and chop.

CRISPY YELLOWTAIL PARMESAN

I should be famous because of this recipe! It's simple but absolutely delicious. Yellowtail snapper is the preferred fish for many native Floridians and tourists. It is sweet, flaky and tender, and when blended with the buttery texture of Parmesan cheese, will literally melt in your mouth. Serve this to your guests, and they'll think you're a culinary genius.

1 pound yellowtail filets
2 Tablespoons butter, melted
2/3 cup seasoned breadcrumbs
1/3 cup fresh Parmesan cheese, finely grated
2 Tablespoons olive oil

Rinse filets and pat dry. Combine breadcrumbs and Parmesan cheese in shallow dish. Apply thin layer of butter to filets and roll in breadcrumb mixture, coating evenly. In large, non-stick skillet, heat olive oil over medium-high heat until hot. Sauté filets 4-6 minutes per side, depending on thickness, until fish is golden brown and crisp. Remove from skillet and serve.

Serves 4.

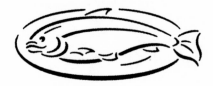

Spice-Rubbed Yellowtail
with
Nectarine Salsa

Yellowtail snapper is such a delicate fish that it doesn't take much effort to enhance its natural flavor and tenderness. Here, we've rubbed filets with a blend of spices paired with a sensational salsa using some of summer's most popular fruits.

For Salsa:
>   1 large nectarine, chopped into ½-inch cubes
>   8 cherry tomatoes, quartered
>   ½ avocado, chopped
>   2 scallions, sliced thin
>   1 jalapeno, seeded and finely chopped
>   3 Tablespoons fresh basil, chopped
>   1 Tablespoon honey
>   1 Tablespoon red wine vinegar
>   1 Tablespoon fresh lime juice
>   ½-1 teaspoon hot sauce

For Fish:
>   1½ pounds yellowtail snapper filets, skinned and boned
>   ½ teaspoon coarse salt
>   1 teaspoon fresh cracked pepper
>   1 teaspoon cumin
>   ½ teaspoon paprika
>   teaspoon garlic powder
>   1/8 teaspoon chili powder
>   1 Tablespoon olive oil

In medium bowl, combine nectarines, cherry tomatoes, avocado, scallions and jalapeno. Add vinegar, honey, lime juice and hot sauce and stir until well blended. Add basil and gently toss to blend. Refrigerate 30 minutes or more. In small bowl, combine salt, pepper, cumin, paprika and garlic powder. Mix well. Rinse filets and pat dry. Rub lightly with olive oil. Rub spice mixture onto yellowtail filets and refrigerate 30 minutes. In large, non-stick skillet, heat 1 Tablespoon olive oil over medium-high heat until hot, but not smoking. Add filets to skillet and pan-sear until golden brown, about 4 minutes per side. Serve with nectarine salsa.

Serves 2-4.

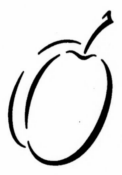

NATIVE SNAPPER WITH FRESH TOMATO, OLIVE AND CAPER SAUCE

Cooking under pressure is my idea of fun. One summer night on our boat in the Bahamas, I challenged myself to come up with a quick and delicious recipe. The sun was setting, mosquitoes were buzzing and the clock was ticking. Using just a few ingredients, I created this simple and quick pan-seared sauce to complement a gently crusted yellowtail snapper. My best advice is to leave plenty of time to savor the results!

For sauce:

2 fresh, vine-ripened tomatoes, seeded and coarsely chopped

¼ cup Calamata olives, pitted and chopped

2 Tablespoons capers

1 Tablespoon white wine vinegar

1 Tablespoon fresh lemon juice

2 Tablespoons fresh parsley, chopped

2 Tablespoons fresh basil, chopped

For fish:

1 pound yellowtail snapper filets, skinned

½ cup all-purpose flour

½ cup Progresso seasoned Italian bread crumbs

Salt and pepper to taste

2 Tablespoons olive oil

In medium bowl, combine sauce ingredients and set aside to marinate. In small, shallow bowl, combine flour and breadcrumbs and set aside. Season fish with salt and pepper, then dredge fish in flour and breadcrumb mixture to coat. (This technique is more like dusting filets with flour than battering them.) Using non-stick skillet, heat olive oil over medium-high heat. When oil is hot, but not smoking, add filets and sauté until golden brown on each side, 3-4 minutes per side. Remove fish and keep warm on platter. Keeping pan hot, add sauce mixture, which should sizzle from heat. Heat sauce, tossing gently 4-5 minutes until heated through and tomatoes begin to release juices. Tomatoes should not be completely softened. Spoon sauce onto fish and serve.

Serves 4.

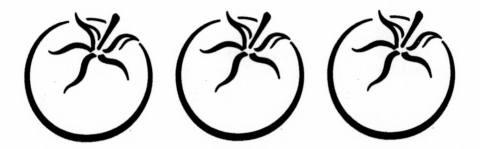

GRILLED MAHI-MAHI
WITH
STIR-FRY VEGETABLES

An exotic blending of Asian flavors enhances the delicate flavor of mahi-mahi, creating an enticing main course. Quick stir-fried vegetables are a colorful complement to the fish, making this light dinner a refreshing change of pace.

For marinade:
   ½ cup sherry
   2 Tablespoons soy sauce
   ½ Tablespoon peanut oil
   1 teaspoon sesame oil
   ¼ cup hoison sauce
   2 Tablespoons scallions, minced
   2 Tablespoons ginger, minced
   ½ teaspoon garlic powder
   Juice of one lime
   ½ cup fresh cilantro, chopped
   Two 6-ounce mahi-mahi filets

For stir fry:
   2 teaspoons peanut oil
   1 cup snow peas, trimmed and cleaned
   1 red bell pepper, seeded and julienned
   4 scallions, sliced
   12 stalks asparagus, cut into 2-inch pieces
   1 can sliced water chestnuts, rinsed and drained
   2 carrots, peeled and julienned
   1 teaspoon sesame oil
   Soy sauce to taste

Combine marinade ingredients and whisk together until well blended. Marinate fish for 1 hour. Remove from marinade and grill until cooked through, about 7 minutes per side. Meanwhile, heat peanut oil in wok and stir-fry vegetables until crisply tender. Add sesame oil and soy sauce to taste. Place vegetables on plate and top with grilled mahi-mahi.

Serves 2.

GRILLED COBIA
WITH
PAPAYA SALSA

Cobia is an extraordinary white fish with a mild flavor and firm texture. It is found primarily off the Florida coast, throughout the Caribbean and in the Gulf of Mexico. Filets are usually cut thick and are excellent for grilling. This recipe offers a simple marinade and a mild fruit salsa to enhance the mellow character of this finned favorite.

For fish:

    1 pound cobia filets
    ¼ cup vegetable oil
    ¼ cup soy sauce
    1 garlic clove, minced
    1 Tablespoon fresh ginger, minced
    2 Tablespoons sesame oil
    Juice of one lime

For salsa:

    ½ cup fresh papaya, cubed
    ¼ cup avocado, cubed
    ½ yellow pepper, chopped
    ½ jalapeno, seeded and minced
    2 scallions, thinly sliced
    1 Tablespoon white wine vinegar
    1 Tablespoon honey
    2 Tablespoons lime juice
    2 Tablespoons fresh orange juice
    2 Tablespoons fresh mint, chopped
    1 Tablespoon fresh, flat-leaf parsley, chopped

Whisk together vegetable oil, soy sauce, garlic, ginger, sesame oil and lime. Place fish in shallow dish and marinate for 1 hour. Combine salsa ingredients and set aside. Grill fish over medium-hot coals until opaque, 6-7 minutes per side. In separate bowl, combine salsa ingredients. Toss well and chill slightly before serving.

Serves 4.

> ***Quick Tip:*** *If you can't find cobia at your market, try swordfish, dolphin, wahoo or monkfish. Cobia is not popular with commercial fishermen because it is not easy to catch. So the general rule of thumb on cobia is: If it is in your market, it should be very fresh, because it was probably caught that day.*

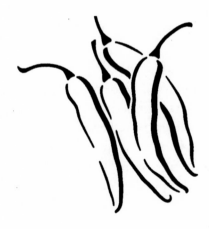

GRILLED TUNA
WITH
PUTTANESCA RELISH

Here's an excellent alternative for tuna steaks. This creation is inspired by the robust flavors of Italy's famous Puttanesca sauce, which is renowned for its simplicity. The tomato and garlic sauce is tangy, rich in flavor and exceptionally satisfying. This relish is also excellent with swordfish steaks. True to its concept, the preparation is simple and the taste is sensational.

Two 6- to 8-ounce tuna steaks, preferably yellowfin or
    sashimi-grade tuna
Coarse salt
Fresh cracked pepper
1 Tablespoon olive oil
2 teaspoons olive oil
1 garlic clove, minced
1 pound plum tomatoes, seeded and coarsely chopped
1 Tablespoon capers, drained
¼ cup Calamata olives, pitted and coarsely chopped
1 Tablespoon red wine vinegar
1 Tablespoon anchovy paste
2 Tablespoons fresh parsley, chopped

Prepare grill. Rub tuna steaks with olive oil, then with salt and pepper. Grill tuna to your preference, about 8 minutes per side for medium rare. (It's advisable to keep center of fish slightly pink.) Heat olive oil in non-stick skillet over medium heat. When oil is warm, add garlic and sauté until fragrant. Add tomatoes, capers, olives, and red wine vinegar and sauté until tomatoes are tender, about 5 minutes. Add anchovy paste and fresh parsley, stirring to dissolve anchovy paste. Cook 5 minutes longer. Remove from heat. Serve sauce on tuna steaks.

Serves 2-4.

> *Quick Tip: When cooking tuna on the grill, remember that it will continue to cook even after it is removed from the heat. So to cook it rare to medium-rare, be certain there is a heavy portion of pink in the center when you remove the tuna from the grill.*

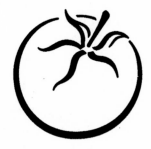

STIR-FRIED MARINATED COBIA

Cobia is an ideal fish for cooking in your wok. Here, I've spiced up the fish and veggie combination, creating a wonderful aromatic balance with fragrant ginger and herbs.

1 pound cobia filets, cut into 2-inch pieces
¼ cup peanut oil
3 Tablespoons light soy sauce
1 Tablespoon fresh ginger, grated
1 garlic clove, minced
3 Tablespoons sherry
½ Tablespoon peanut oil
1 additional Tablespoon light soy sauce
½ cup mushrooms, sliced
2 carrots, sliced diagonally
½ bunch asparagus, cut into 2-inch pieces
½ cup snow peas or green beans, trimmed
4 cups fresh spinach, washed and dried
½ Tablespoon sesame oil
1/3 cup fresh cilantro, chopped

Place cobia pieces in shallow dish or bowl. Combine next 5 ingredients in bowl and whisk vigorously until blended. Pour marinade over fish and marinate 1 hour. Remove from marinade and drain thoroughly. In wok, heat ½ Tablespoon peanut oil until hot and just smoking. Add fish and stir fry, tossing or turning frequently for about 8 minutes, until cooked through. Remove fish from wok and keep warm. In same wok, add mushrooms, carrots, asparagus and snow peas and toss to coat with remaining oil. Add remaining 1 Tablespoon soy sauce and toss again. Cook 1-2 minutes, add spinach and toss until it begins to wilt. Drizzle with sesame oil. Continue tossing until spinach is just wilted and vegetables are crisply tender. Remove from heat. Serve vegetables on plates and top with fish. Sprinkle with cilantro.

Serves 4.

HERB-SEALED GROUPER ON THE GRILL

Mention the word "grouper" to most Floridians and their mouths will water! Grouper would definitely win the popularity contest for fish among locals and tourists. Fortunately, grouper is available in most markets, and this recipe makes it easy to enjoy. This flavorful fish is smothered with beautiful peppers, tomatoes and herbs, then sealed tightly and grilled. The result is a tender fish, steaming with herb-infused flavor.

1 pound grouper filets
1 Vidalia onion, coarsely chopped
2 red peppers, coarsely chopped
1 jalapeno pepper, finely chopped
2 tomatoes, seeded and coarsely chopped
6 sprigs fresh thyme
½ cup fresh basil, chopped
6 large green olives, sliced
2 Tablespoons rice vinegar
1teaspoon coarse salt
1 teaspoon fresh cracked pepper

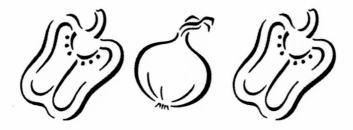

Prepare your grill. Rinse grouper filets and pat dry. On large piece of aluminum foil flattened on work surface, spread peppers, onions and jalapeno in layer equaling size of filets. (If necessary, separate grouper into 2 pieces and arrange on 2 pieces of foil.) Place filets on top of pepper and onion mixture and sprinkle with salt and pepper to taste. Spread tomatoes over grouper, lay thyme sprigs on top and sprinkle with basil. Put olives on top and drizzle with rice vinegar. Wrap foil around seasoned filets and seal air-tight. Place foil packages on grill and cook for 8 minutes (juices will bubble and try to escape packages). Carefully remove from grill and let steam for 1 or 2 minutes. Open foil carefully and serve.

Serves 4-6.

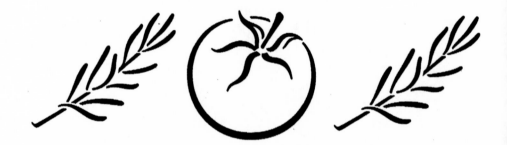

ROASTED RED PEPPER SHRIMP
AND
BLACK BEAN BARBECUE

Here is a delicious new twist for barbecue sauce. Smoky roasted red peppers and a traditional barbecue baste join forces to give this dish a lively personality. The depth of flavor from the peppers adds a new dimension to tender, pan-seared shrimp and hearty black beans. If you have leftovers of this outstanding sauce, use it as a marvelous baste for chicken or pork.

For sauce:
   1 Tablespoon olive oil
   1 clove garlic, minced
   1 medium Vidalia onion, finely chopped
   1 (12-ounce) jar roasted red peppers, drained, rinsed and
      coarsely chopped
   1 jalapeno pepper, seeded and minced
   2 Tablespoons light brown sugar
   1 Tablespoon molasses
   1 Tablespoon Worcestershire sauce
   12 ounces chili sauce
   2 Tablespoons Dijon mustard
   1 Tablespoon Tiger Sauce or hot sauce of your choice

For shrimp and black beans:
   1 Tablespoon olive oil
   1 pound large shrimp, shelled, deveined and cleaned
   1 red pepper, coarsely chopped
   1 jalapeno pepper, minced, with seeds removed
   1 (15-ounce) can black beans, rinsed and drained
   1 cup cooked fresh corn kernels (or frozen and thawed)
   ¼ red onion, diced
   ¼ cup fresh cilantro, chopped

First make sauce. In medium-sized saucepan, heat olive oil with garlic and onion over medium heat until translucent. Add peppers and sauté until just tender, about 4 minutes. Add brown sugar, molasses, Worcestershire, chili sauce, Dijon mustard and Tiger Sauce and stir to blend. Simmer over medium-low heat for 15 minutes. Remove from heat and let sauce cool to room temperature. Heat oil in heavy, deep skillet over medium heat. Add shrimp, red pepper and jalapeno and cook until shrimp are just pink, about 5 minutes. Reduce heat to low and simmer for 2 more minutes. Add beans, corn and red onion and stir until heated through, about 2 minutes. Add ¼ cup barbecue sauce and stir thoroughly to heat through, about 5 minutes. Serve over rice and garnish with cilantro. Serve extra barbecue sauce on side.

Serves 4.

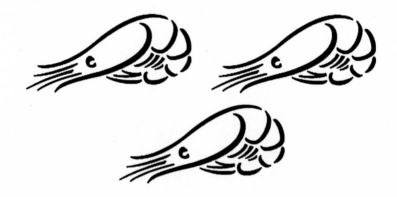

LEMON DILL SHRIMP SAUTÉ

Quick, snappy and packed with flavor, this is one of most expedient dinners you will ever make. Scallions lend their assertive character to this dish, while fresh dill gives it a distinctive edge. Serve it with your favorite rice pilaf or a side of simple pasta, and you will have an exceptional meal.

1 pound large shrimp, shelled and deveined
1 bunch scallions, sliced on diagonal into 1-inch pieces
1 Tablespoon butter
1 Tablespoon olive oil
1 Tablespoon fresh dill, chopped, or 1½ teaspoons dried
    dill
2 Tablespoons lemon juice
Fresh ground pepper
Salt to taste

In large, non-stick skillet, heat butter and olive oil over medium heat. Add scallions and sauté until just softened, about 4 minutes. Add shrimp and cook about 5 minutes, stirring often to cook through. When shrimp are just turning pink, add lemon juice, dill and pepper and toss together. Cook 2 more minutes until sauce is slightly thickened and shrimp are coated. Remove from heat and serve.

Serves 2-4.

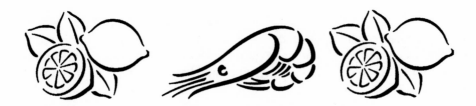

TROPICAL SHRIMP RISOTTO

Lucky for us, Florida is abundant with shrimp. From Key West pink to white or brown, all of which are caught off the coast, shrimp is a favorite seafood of both visitors and residents. Here, a combination of tropical fruit complements this tender shellfish, creating a risotto-style rice dish with extraordinary flavors.

1½ cups basmati rice
3½ cups vegetable broth (use low-sodium broth, if you
    can find it)
½ Tablespoon butter
1 Tablespoon olive oil
1 yellow onion, minced
1 garlic clove, minced
1¼ pounds medium shrimp, shelled and deveined
¼ cup fresh basil, chopped
½ cup dry white wine
1 mango, chopped into 1-inch dice
1 cup fresh pineapple, chopped into 1-inch dice
2 Tablespoons cornstarch
Juice of one large lemon
½ cup orange juice
1 teaspoon orange rind
2 teaspoons curry powder
2 Tablespoons brown sugar

In medium saucepan, bring vegetable broth to boil and add rice and butter. Reduce heat to medium-low and simmer 20-25 minutes, until liquid is absorbed. In large saucepan, sauté onion and garlic in olive oil until soft. Add shrimp and sauté until just pink. Add white wine and basil and stir. Add mango and pineapple, cover and sauté 10 minutes. In separate bowl, mix cornstarch with lemon juice, orange juice, orange rind, curry and brown sugar, stirring until well blended. Add sauce to shrimp and fruit mixture and stir until mixture is thickened and sauce coats shrimp and fruit. Add rice to shrimp and fruit mixture and stir until all ingredients are coated with sauce. Simmer 8 minutes to blend flavors. Garnish with fresh basil and serve.

Serves 4-6.

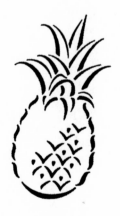

PAN-SEARED COLOSSAL SHRIMP
WITH
CRANBERRY ORANGE SALSA

Here is a festive salsa that is superb for entertaining during the holidays. The colors are vibrant and the citrus flavors are welcoming. Shrimp may not be traditional holiday cuisine, but this recipe with its brilliant and tasty salsa is worth breaking tradition. Be sure to buy jumbo/colossal shrimp, sometimes known as "prawns."

> 1 cup water
> 1 cup sugar
> 2 cups whole cranberries (fresh or frozen), rinsed and picked through
> 2 cinnamon sticks
> One 2-inch piece fresh ginger, peeled and sliced into ¼-inch pieces
> ½ unpeeled orange, quartered
> 1 orange, peeled and diced, with seeds removed
> 1 shallot, minced
> ½ red pepper, diced
> 3 Tablespoons golden raisins
> 2 Tablespoons sherry vinegar
> 1 Tablespoon walnut oil
> 1 Tablespoon Grand Marnier liqueur
> 2 pounds jumbo/colossal shrimp, peeled and deveined
> 2 Tablespoons olive oil

Bring water to boil and add cranberries, sugar, cinnamon, ginger and unpeeled orange halves. Simmer 10 minutes over low heat until cranberries are slightly softened, but still holding their shape. Remove from heat. Remove orange pieces with slotted spoon and discard. Cool mixture slightly. In medium-sized bowl, combine peeled and diced orange pieces, shallot, red pepper and raisins. After cranberry mixture cools, use slotted spoon to remove cinnamon sticks and transfer cranberries to bowl with diced orange pieces, draining off as much liquid as possible. Reserve liquid. Add 2 Tablespoons reserved syrup from cranberry mixture. Add vinegar, walnut oil and Grand Marnier and stir to combine. Set salsa aside and prepare shrimp. In large, non-stick skillet, heat olive oil over medium-high heat. Sauté shrimp until pink and cooked through, 3-4 minutes per side. Serve shrimp on plate with salsa in center.

Serves 4-6.

CORNMEAL-CRUSTED SHRIMP
WITH
JALAPENO JELLY

If you are a fried shrimp lover, but have abandoned fried foods, you will adore this recipe! Spicy cornmeal coating gives this shrimp a golden, crunchy crust. Jalapeno jelly, which is available at most gourmet markets, adds a sweet, spicy kick.

> 1½ pounds (15-18 count) extra-large shrimp, shelled and
>   deveined
> 2/3 cup corn meal
> 4 scallions, finely minced
> ½ teaspoon garlic powder
> Dash of black pepper
> 2 egg whites, lightly beaten with 1 Tablespoon water
> 2 Tablespoons olive oil
> ¼ cup jalapeno jelly*

*Available at many supermarkets and gourmet markets.

In shallow dish, combine cornmeal, scallions, garlic powder and black pepper and combine well. Place lightly beaten egg whites in shallow bowl. Dip shrimp in egg whites and coat on both sides, then dip into cornmeal mixture and coat completely. In skillet, heat olive oil over medium-high heat. Place shrimp in skillet and cook until crisp and golden brown, 5-7 minutes on each side. Serve with jalapeno jelly.

Serves 4.

Variations:

Other sauces to try with this recipe:
Pink Tartar Sauce
Apricot Horseradish Sauce
Traditional Cocktail Sauce

SHRIMP PASTA WITH MUSHROOMS
AND
SUN-DRIED TOMATOES

This lively pasta creation is a delicious, light entree that can be prepared in no time. The intriguing blend of mushrooms and artichoke hearts adds richness to the shrimp, and the sun-dried tomatoes give it a satisfying, robust flavor.

    1 Tablespoon olive oil
    1 clove garlic, minced
    ¼ teaspoon dried red pepper flakes
    1 pound large shrimp, peeled and deveined
    2 cups mixed mushrooms such as crimini, shiitake, button and
        oyster, sliced
    ¾ cup marinated artichoke hearts, drained and quartered
    ½ cup sun-dried tomatoes, softened in boiling water
    ½ cup white wine
    ¼ cup clam juice or vegetable broth
    ¼ cup fresh basil, chopped
    ¼ cup fresh oregano, chopped
    Salt and pepper to taste
    4 ounces fresh Parmesan cheese, grated

In non-stick skillet, heat olive oil over medium-high heat until warm. Add red pepper flakes and garlic, stirring until fragrant. Add shrimp and sauté until just cooked through and pink. Remove from skillet, set aside and keep warm. To skillet, add mushrooms, artichoke hearts and sun-dried tomatoes. Sauté for 5 minutes until mushrooms are tender. Add white wine or broth and simmer until slightly reduced, about 5 minutes. Meanwhile, cook pasta al dente. Drain thoroughly. Add shrimp to mushroom and artichoke heart mixture and toss until heated through. Add basil, oregano, salt and pepper to taste, and keep warm. Add pasta to skillet, and toss. Sprinkle with grated Parmesan cheese.

Serves 4.

Quick Tip: Pasta Tricks: To keep pasta from becoming dry or sticky, try the following tricks:

- *After cooking, drain pasta and toss with 1 Tablespoon olive oil*
- *Add up to ¼ cup additional vegetable broth, white wine or reserved pasta water to your sauce just before serving*
- *Drizzle the pasta with hot pasta water just before tossing with your sauce*

DAD'S BEST BROILED LOBSTER TAILS
WITH
HERB BUTTER

My dad does not spend a lot of time in the kitchen, but he has passed along this flawless recipe and procedure for preparing lobster tails. Dad is a native Miamian, so he has eaten his share of lobster. In this recipe, lobster is broiled to tender perfection and basted with delicious herb butter. There's no doubt, my dad knows best when it comes to this delicious crustacean!

4 Florida lobster tails, split
½ cup clarified butter
3 Tablespoons chives, chopped
1 Tablespoon lime zest
½ teaspoon red pepper flakes
1 teaspoon Asian chili sauce
3 Tablespoons fresh cilantro or basil, chopped
1 Tablespoon fresh lime juice

Preheat broiler and place oven rack on second-highest level. In small saucepan used to clarify butter, combine chives, zest, pepper flakes, chili sauce, lime juice and cilantro or basil over low heat and stir well. Keep over low heat for 10-15 minutes, while preparing lobster tails. Broil tails, shell side up, for 6 minutes on rack with oven door closed. Turn lobster tails over and place meat side up. Brush liberally with herb butter. Return to broiler for 8 minutes, with oven door partially open. Use remaining melted butter for dipping.

Serves 4.

> *Quick Tip: To clarify butter, melt over low heat and simmer until it starts to foam. Remove from heat. Using spoon, skim foam off top and discard. Butter should be as close to clear as possible.*

BEER-BATTERED BAHAMIAN CRAWFISH

The smell and taste of beer batter takes me back to my childhood. Dad would come home from a day of fishing, and we would patiently wait for Mom to fry his fresh catch in a crispy, light crust. I don't fry very often these days, but when I do, beer batter, with its tempura-like texture, is my first choice. In this version, I have applied the same cooking method to lobster tails. The key is to get the oil as hot as possible, which will create a crisp coating, and seal in all the fantastic flavor of this luscious shellfish.

> 1 pound lobster-tail meat, shelled and cut into 2-inch pieces
> 1 cup self-rising flour
> ¾ cup beer (if possible, do not use light beer)
> ½ teaspoon fresh ground pepper
> ½ teaspoon salt
> ½ teaspoon garlic and herb seasoning
> 3 cups peanut oil for frying

In large bowl, mix flour with seasonings. Add beer slowly to avoid foaming, and stir to blend. Batter should be slightly thicker than pancake batter. In large, deep pot or deep fryer, heat peanut oil to 350 degrees. (Use fat or candy thermometer, or test oil by dropping one small spoonful of batter into oil. Batter should drop to bottom, then pop up to surface. If you do not see frying action, wait a few more minutes and try again.) Dip several pieces of lobster at a time into batter and drop into hot oil. Fry 3-4 minutes or until golden, then remove from pot and place on plate lined with paper towels. Continue with remaining lobster pieces. When finished, season with salt and pepper, and serve with Pink Tartar Sauce or Apricot Horseradish Sauce.

Serves 4.

> *Quick Tip: To remove tail meat from lobster, use large, sharp knife to cut tail in half, lengthwise. Use fingers to peel meat away from shell in one piece.*

SWEET PEPPERED SCALLOPS

Sweet, tender bay scallops and a variety of pleasantly pungent peppers blend together in this main course that is as easy to prepare as it is to devour. The fun part of this recipe is that you can make it as spicy as you like, with your own blend of chilies such as serranos, scotch bonnets or poblanos. Either way, prepare yourself for a mouth-watering delight.

Non-stick spray
2 teaspoons olive oil
1 red bell pepper, diced
1 yellow bell pepper, diced
½ green bell pepper, diced
1 jalapeno pepper, seeded and minced
4 scallions, sliced
1 pound bay scallops, rinsed and drained
Juice of 1 lemon
3 Tablespoons fresh basil, chopped
Salt and pepper to taste

In non-stick skillet sprayed with non-stick spray, heat olive oil over medium-high heat. Add red, yellow and green peppers, jalapeno and scallions, and sauté until softened, about 5 minutes. Add bay scallops and lemon juice, reduce heat to medium-low and sauté until scallops are translucent. Add basil and salt and pepper to taste. Stir until herbs are fragrant, about 3 minutes.

Serves 2-4.

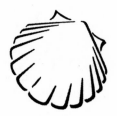

Quick Tip on Chilies: Peppers are widely known as "chilies," and there is usually a good selection to choose from at most markets. Rating them from 1 to 10, with 10 being the hottest, here are the varieties that would work best in this recipe:

Jalapeno is a popular, fiery pepper that is very palatable in most recipes. Named for the Mexican capital of Veracruz, it gives a peppery kick without setting your mouth on fire. (7-8 rating)

Serrano peppers are as hot as jalapenos, but have a sharper taste. (7-8 rating)

Scotch Bonnet is among hottest of chilies and has a citrus flavor. They turn from green to yellow and then to red and increase in heat as they ripen. (10 rating)

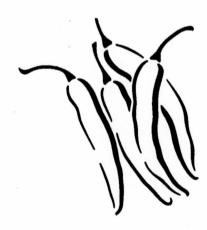

PAN-SEARED SCALLOPS
WITH
PAPAYA YELLOW TOMATO SALSA

This sunset-colored salsa provides the perfect backdrop for the distinctive natural flavor of sea scallops. Yellow tomatoes are low in acid and have a mild taste that complements the mellow sweetness of papaya. If you can't find yellow tomatoes, use cherry tomatoes or the best vine-red ones you can find.

For salsa:
    ½ cup papaya, diced
    1 yellow tomato, seeded and diced
    ½ red bell pepper, chopped
    1 jalapeno, minced
    3 scallions, chopped
    1 Tablespoon lime zest
    1 teaspoon honey
    1 Tablespoon lime juice
    3 Tablespoons red wine vinegar

For scallops:
    1 pound sea scallops
    1 Tablespoon olive oil
    1 teaspoon sea salt
    1 teaspoon pepper
    ¼ teaspoon ground white pepper

For salsa: Combine all ingredients in medium bowl and chill one hour.

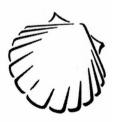

For scallops: Rinse scallops and pat dry with paper towel. Season both sides with salt, pepper and white pepper. Heat olive oil in large, non-stick skillet over medium-high heat. When oil is hot, but not smoking, place scallops in pan and cook about 2 minutes per side until lightly golden. Serve with salsa.

Serves 4.

Quick Tip: I admit I am a major papaya fan! I envy my neighbors who have papaya trees in their backyards. Papaya grown in Florida are sweet and fragrant. I became hooked on papaya on a trip to Hawaii, and am always searching the markets for the ripest, sweetest fruit. So, how can you tell if a papaya is ripe? The skin should be turning from green to yellow-orange. There may be some pock marks or irregularities, and the fruit should have a subtly sweet smell. When you slice it in half, the flesh should be a bright orange. Remove seeds and peel skin with sharp knife, then proceed with recipe directions.

PAN-SEARED SEA SCALLOPS
WITH
CITRUS REDUCTION

Scallops are definitely one of Mother Ocean's greatest gifts. Bay, sea and calico scallops are abundant in the Gulf of Mexico and along Florida's northern coast. In this recipe, large, tender scallops are seared to seal in flavor, then complemented with a sauce that draws extra body and tartness from a blend of apricot and citrus.

1 pound sea scallops
Coarse salt
Fresh black pepper
Garlic and herb seasoning
1 Tablespoon olive oil
2 shallots, chopped
1 Tablespoon butter
2 Tablespoons red wine vinegar
½ cup clam juice
½ cup fresh orange juice
3 sprigs fresh thyme
1 Tablespoon orange zest
3 Tablespoons apricot preserves
½ teaspoon cornstarch mixed with 1 Tablespoon water
2 Tablespoons Half-and-Half
2 Tablespoons fresh thyme, chopped

Brush grill pan with olive oil and heat over medium-high heat. Season scallops with garlic and herb seasoning, salt and pepper. When pan is hot, sear scallops about 3-4 minutes per side until golden and crusty. Remove from pan and keep warm. In another skillet, heat butter over medium-high heat and add shallots. Sauté until shallots are tender, add vinegar and stir until slightly reduced. Add orange juice and clam juice to mixture and bring to simmer. Add thyme sprigs and orange zest and simmer about 8 minutes, until liquid is reduced to 1/3 cup. Strain sauce in sieve and return to skillet. Add preserves and stir until smooth. Add ½ cornstarch mixture and stir until thickened. Remove from heat and whisk in Half-and-Half, stirring until blended. Season with salt and pepper to taste. To serve, spoon sauce onto plates and top with scallops. Garnish with minced fresh thyme. Serve with fragrant basmati or jasmine rice.

Serves 2-4.

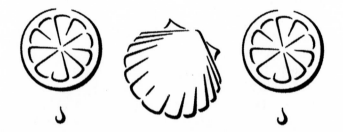

SKINNY CRAB
AND
ASPARAGUS QUICHE

Here is an updated, modified quiche loaded with healthful, tasty ingredients. This quiche has no crust and resembles a frittata. You can serve this tasty, low-fat and incredibly versatile dish for brunch, for lunch or as a light dinner!

1 cup lump crab meat, rinsed and picked over to remove shells
1 teaspoon olive oil
¾ cup fresh white button mushrooms, sliced
4 scallions, sliced on diagonal in 1-inch pieces
½ pound asparagus, sliced on diagonal in 1-inch pieces and blanched
4 ounces, light Jarlsberg cheese, shredded
¾ cup low-fat cottage cheese
3 Tablespoons white wine
3 eggs
1 Tablespoon fresh parsley
½ teaspoon salt
½ teaspoon fresh cracked pepper
2 teaspoons Dijon mustard

Preheat oven to 375. Spray 9-inch tart pan or pie plate with non-stick coating. Pat crabmeat dry and spread on bottom of pie plate. In non-stick skillet, heat olive oil over medium-high heat and add mushrooms and scallions. Sauté until tender and cool slightly. Transfer mushrooms and scallions to pie plate and spread on top of crabmeat. Layer blanched asparagus and shredded cheese. In blender, whirl together cottage cheese, wine, eggs, salt, pepper and Dijon mustard. Pour over layered ingredients in pie plate. Bake for 45-50 minutes or until firm and set.

Serves 6.

> *Quick Tip:* To blanch asparagus: Clean and trim asparagus, bring medium pot of water to boil, drop asparagus into boiling water and cook for 2 minutes. Drain and rinse in cold water. Transfer to bowl of ice water to stop the cooking process. If using pencil-thin asparagus, reduce cooking time by 30 seconds.

> *Variation:* Make this a traditional quiche by simply adding the crust. Follow the same directions, but place the ingredients into an unbaked, prepared pie crust.

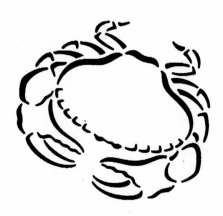

Chapter 4

From the Land

Grilled Chicken Pasta Salad with Light Peanut Dressing
Grilled Mambo Chicken with Red Pepper Coulis
Grilled Jamaican Chicken Salad with Honey Dijon Vinaigrette
Mango Barbecue Chicken
Pepita Cornmeal-Crusted Chicken with Herbed Goat Cheese
and Essence of Dried Cranberries
Tequila-Spiked Turkey Pepper Chili
Farm Fresh Fajitas with Seasoned Black Beans
Cross Creek Ajiaco
Penne Primavera with Feta
Asian Stir-Fry Pasta
Plum Tomato Pasta
Mediterranean Penne Pasta
Pasta with Chicken, Fennel and Sun-dried Tomatoes
Alfresco Tomato Arugula Pasta
Light-Heavyweight Champion Pasta
Red Wine-Infused Beef Kabobs
Bourbon Balsamic Barbecue Pork Tenderloin
Skillet-Seared Lamb Chops with Lemon, Artichokes and Dill
Classic Veal Piccata

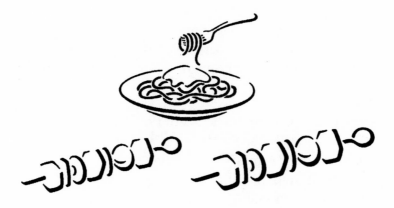

GRILLED CHICKEN PASTA SALAD
WITH
LIGHT PEANUT DRESSING

This recipe captures the wonderful decadence of an Asian peanut sauce. There are a few tricks here that help to cut fat and calories while retaining richness and texture. Tossed with a colorful array of vegetables and smoky grilled chicken, this dish can be served at room temperature, which makes it a great choice for outdoor entertaining.

For Salad:
>½ pound tricolor fusilli
>½ Tablespoon peanut oil
>1 cup asparagus, chopped into 1-inch pieces
>2 carrots, julienned
>1 red pepper, julienned
>1 medium stalk celery, cleaned and sliced crosswise
>½ cup seedless cucumber, peeled and julienned
>2 boneless, skinless chicken breasts, cleaned and trimmed
>Coarse salt
>Fresh cracked pepper
>Garlic and herb seasoning
>4 scallions, sliced on diagonal
>3 Tablespoons unsalted, dry-roasted peanuts
>½ cup fresh cilantro, chopped

For dressing:
>3 Tablespoons reduced-fat peanut butter
>3 Tablespoons boiling water
>¼ cup coconut rum or coconut liqueur
>¼ cup skim milk or light coconut milk
>3 Tablespoons reduced-sodium soy sauce
>½ Tablespoon sesame oil

2 teaspoons hot sauce
1 Tablespoon lime zest
3 Tablespoons fresh lime juice
½ teaspoon salt
1 Tablespoon fresh ginger, minced
1 clove garlic, minced

Prepare grill. Season chicken breasts with salt, pepper and garlic and herb seasoning. Grill chicken until cooked through to desired doneness. Bring large pot of water to boil. Drop in asparagus and cook 1-2 minutes or until it turns bright green. Transfer to bowl of ice water. Drop carrots in boiling water for 1-2 minutes and transfer to same bowl. When carrots and asparagus are chilled, drain, pat dry and set aside. In same pot of boiling water, cook pasta al dente. Rinse with cold water to prevent sticking. In bowl, combine pasta, carrots, asparagus, celery, red pepper and cucumber.

For dressing: In medium bowl, combine peanut butter with hot water, pouring in a stream and stirring constantly until mixture is smooth. Add coconut rum and skim milk and stir again, until smooth. Add soy sauce, sesame oil, lime juice and lime zest and stir until well blended. Add salt, ginger and garlic and stir well. Toss salad with sauce until well coated. Add cooked chicken and scallions and toss again. Sprinkle with cilantro and peanuts and serve.

Serves 4-6 as main course, 8-10 as side dish.

GRILLED MAMBO CHICKEN
WITH
RED PEPPER COULIS

It's almost impossible to avoid Latin influences in Florida, and who would want to? South Florida has become a dynamic melting pot of Central and South American culture and culinary diversity. Whether they are from Cuba, Mexico, Colombia, Venezuela or Ecuador, our new residents inspire us to embrace their upbeat and colorful style. This particular culinary creation reflects the spirit and character of Latin cuisine. So play your favorite Latin tunes, practice your salsa steps and get ready for some lively flavors!

1 (15-ounce) can black beans, rinsed and drained
1/3 cup or more white wine
1 clove garlic, minced
1 Tablespoon Tiger Sauce (or hot sauce of your choice)
1 Tablespoon olive oil, plus 2 teaspoons
1 jalapeno pepper, seeded and chopped
1 teaspoon cumin
2 cups roasted red peppers (about 4 peppers, total)
½ teaspoon chili powder
1 Tablespoon white wine vinegar
2 teaspoons cracked black pepper
2 teaspoons coarsely ground salt
2 whole, skinless chicken breasts, halved, trimmed and
    pounded to ½-inch thickness
Juice of 1 lime
1 bunch (6) fresh scallions, with tips trimmed and 1/3 of
    green ends cut off
¼ cup fresh cilantro
2 red peppers, halved and seeded and cut into ½-inch
    strips

For puree:

Combine ¾ can black beans, ¼ cup white wine, garlic, ½ Tablespoon olive oil, ½ teaspoon cumin, jalapeno and hot sauce in food processor or blender and puree until smooth. Transfer to sauce pan and warm over medium heat. Add remaining black beans to black bean sauce with lime juice and white wine. Stir until smooth and heated through.

For red-pepper coulis:

In food processor or blender, combine 2 cups roasted peppers with chili powder, 1/2 teaspoon cumin, 2 teaspoons olive oil and white wine vinegar. Puree until smooth. Strain through sieve into small saucepan and keep warm. Season to taste with salt and pepper.

For chicken:

Heat remaining ½ Tablespoon olive oil over medium-high heat, in non-stick grill pan sprayed with non-stick spray or prepare your grill. Sprinkle chicken breasts with salt and pepper and rub lightly into chicken. When oil is hot, but not smoking, place chicken in skillet and sear both sides until almost cooked through, about 5 minutes per side. Or, grill chicken breasts over medium-hot fire until done, about 6 minutes per side.

For peppers and scallions:

In grill pan, reduce heat to medium. Add scallions and red peppers. Sauté until tender and lightly charred. Remove from pan. On grill, roast red peppers until lightly charred and grill scallions for 1-2 minutes per side. Remove from grill and keep warm.

To serve:

Spoon mambo sauce onto half of plate and spoon red pepper coulis decoratively on other half. Top with chicken, grilled red peppers and scallions, and garnish with cilantro.

Serves 4.

GRILLED JAMAICAN CHICKEN SALAD
WITH
HONEY DIJON VINAIGRETTE

This dish is fiery hot, subtly sweet and guaranteed to light up your taste buds. Jamaican seasonings are known for their gusto, and this main course salad has plenty. Serve it with your favorite corn bread and a cold Red Stripe beer, and you'll find yourself relaxing Jamaica-style!

For dressing:
    1 Tablespoon honey mustard
    1 Tablespoon Dijon mustard
    2 Tablespoons white wine vinegar
    1 Tablespoon lemon juice
    2 teaspoons horseradish
    2 Tablespoons honey
    2 Tablespoons olive oil
    1 Tablespoon plain yogurt
    1 Tablespoon fresh tarragon, chopped

For jerk marinade:
    ½ small onion, finely chopped
    ¼ cup scallions, finely chopped
    2 teaspoons fresh thyme
    1 teaspoon ground allspice
    ¼ teaspoon nutmeg
    ½ teaspoon ground cinnamon
    4 jalapeno peppers, seeded and minced
    1 teaspoon black pepper
    1 Tablespoon fresh ginger, finely grated
    1 Tablespoon Worcestershire sauce
    1 Tablespoon soy sauce
    1 Tablespoon red wine vinegar

For salad:

    2 boneless, skinless chicken breasts

    4 cups mixed lettuce (romaine, arugula, radicchio, endive)

    2 nectarines, sliced into ½-inch wedges

    1 yellow pepper, sliced thin, lengthwise

    6 button mushrooms, sliced

    2 ounces Jarlsberg cheese, grated

    1/3 cup toasted, salted pumpkin seeds

In medium bowl, combine first 6 ingredients for dressing and whisk together. Add oil and yogurt and whisk vigorously until emulsified. In medium bowl, mix ingredients together to make jerk marinade paste. Use food processor with steel blade, if needed. (Stores for up to 1 month in refrigerator.)

Use about 2 Tablespoons of jerk seasoning and rub sparingly over chicken breast until covered. Cover and refrigerate about 30 minutes. Grill chicken over medium fire until cooked through, 8 minutes per side. In large salad bowl, combine lettuce, peppers, mushrooms and cheese and toss with dressing. Serve salad onto plates and top with chicken, nectarines and pumpkin seeds. Drizzle 1 additional Tablespoon of dressing over salads and serve.

Serves 4.

Quick Tip: If you are short on time, use purchased Jamaican jerk marinade and your favorite commercial brand of honey mustard dressing.

MANGO BARBECUE CHICKEN

Mangos are known as the "fruit of paradise," which is appropriate since they are grown throughout the tropics and Latin America. There are numerous varieties of mangoes, but my favorites are Haden, Edwards, Kent and Keitt, which bloom until late September. During their season, mangoes are so abundant that I use them often when experimenting with new recipes such as this one. Here is a uniquely sweet and tangy barbecue sauce that makes an excellent baste for grilled chicken.

1 mango, peeled and pitted
¼ cup fresh-squeezed orange juice
3 Tablespoons rice wine vinegar
2 Tablespoons soy sauce
1 Tablespoon molasses
1 Tablespoon brown sugar
3 scallions, chopped
2 Tablespoons fresh cilantro, chopped
1 Tablespoon Tiger Sauce
Juice of one lime
¼ cup rum
1½ pounds boneless, skinless chicken breasts.

In food processor or blender, puree mango with orange juice, vinegar, soy sauce, molasses and brown sugar until smooth. Add Tiger Sauce (or other hot sauce), scallions, cilantro, lime juice and rum and puree using pulsing motion. Sauce will be slightly chunky. Prepare grill. Grill chicken breasts over medium-high heat. Baste with mango barbecue sauce in last 3 minutes of grill time to prevent burning. Reserve extra sauce to serve on side.

Serves 4.

Quick Tip: How do you know if a mango is ripe? First, check the color. The skin should be orange-red. Second, smell the fruit; it should be fragrant. Third, it should yield slightly to gentle pressure. Mangoes ripen quickly, so use them right away.

PEPITA CORNMEAL-CRUSTED CHICKEN WITH HERBED GOAT CHEESE AND ESSENCE OF DRIED CRANBERRIES

Pepitas (also known as green pumpkin seeds) are an under-utilized delicacy. Flavorful, nutritionally valuable and possessing a great texture, they have gained popularity in both Latin and New World cooking circles. This sophisticated, but uncomplicated entree features a crisp coating of cornmeal and pepitas, a sinful filling of herbed goat cheese and the elegant essence of cranberries.

For chicken and stuffing:
- 4 chicken breast cutlets or skinless, boneless chicken breasts pounded with a mallet to ½-inch thickness
- ½ cup toasted, salted pumpkin seeds, ground medium-fine
- ¼ cup corn meal
- ½ cup buttermilk
- 6 ounces goat cheese
- 2 Tablespoons fresh rosemary, chopped
- 2 Tablespoons fresh thyme, chopped
- 1 Tablespoon butter at room temperature
- 3 Tablespoons scallions, minced
- 1 garlic clove, minced
- ¼ teaspoon white pepper

For sauce:
- 1 shallot, minced
- 2 Tablespoons butter
- 1 cup dry white wine
- ½ cup reduced-sodium chicken broth
- 1 teaspoon balsamic vinegar
- 5 sprigs fresh thyme
- ½ cup dried cranberries
- ½ cup whole cranberry sauce

Fresh cracked pepper to taste

Preheat oven to 400 degrees. With fork, mix goat cheese, butter, rosemary, thyme, scallion, garlic and pepper and set aside. Mix pumpkin seeds and cornmeal and place mixture in shallow dish. Put buttermilk in medium bowl. Prepare chicken breast cutlets or skinless, boneless chicken breasts, finishing with 4 large, flat (½-inch thick) pieces. Spread goat cheese mixture equally in center of each piece and fold in half. Dip each piece in buttermilk and roll in pumpkin seed and cornmeal mixture until well coated. Place in baking dish sprayed with non-stick cooking spray and bake in preheated oven for 40 minutes.

While chicken bakes, prepare sauce as follows: In heavy skillet, melt 1 Tablespoon butter over medium heat. Add shallots and sauté until tender, about 8 minutes. Add wine, chicken stock, balsamic vinegar and fresh thyme sprigs and simmer over medium-low heat until reduced by half, about 15 minutes. Strain mixture in sieve and return sauce to skillet. Add dried cranberries and 1 Tablespoon butter and stir until butter is melted. Add whole cranberry sauce and continue stirring to blend. Keep sauce warm. To serve, place chicken on plates and spoon on sauce.

Serves 4.

TEQUILA-SPIKED TURKEY PEPPER CHILI

This hearty main course is packed with wholesome ingredients and dynamic flavors that will satisfy any appetite. It also lends itself to a wide range of entertaining options. Make it for an easy weeknight dinner or a football party, or heat it up on a cool winter evening. Serve it with your favorite cornbread and you will have a feast. Try to buy fresh ground turkey breast; the quality of flavor will make a difference.

1 pound ground turkey breast
1 teaspoon olive oil
½ large onion, chopped
½ red bell pepper, chopped
½ green bell pepper, chopped
1 jalapeno pepper, seeded and chopped
1 Tablespoon chili powder
1 teaspoon cumin
½ teaspoon cinnamon
1 garlic clove, minced
2 cups chopped canned tomatoes
1/3 cup tomato sauce
¼ cup tequila
1 (7-ounce) can green chilies, chopped
1 (16-ounce) can black beans, rinsed and drained
1 cup kidney beans, rinsed and drained
12 small green olives, coarsely chopped
¼ cup fresh cilantro, chopped
Sour cream (optional)

In large pot, heat olive oil over medium heat. Add onion and garlic and sauté until tender. Add ground turkey and cook until just done, about 7 minutes. Drain excess liquid. Add peppers and sauté until just tender, 2-3 minutes. Add chili powder, cumin and cinnamon and stir until fragrant and all ingredients are coated with spices. Add tomatoes, tomato sauce and tequila and stir. Bring to boil and simmer for 15 minutes. Add beans, olives and cilantro and stir. Simmer until heated through, 3-4 minutes. Serve with additional cilantro and dollop of sour cream.

Serves 4-6.

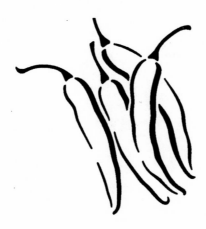

FARM FRESH FAJITAS
WITH
SEASONED BLACK BEANS

There aren't many main courses that bring as much conversation and fun to the dinner table as fajitas. At our family dinners, you would think that fajita-making was a new art form, with someone always claiming to have the best wrapping or folding technique. Of course, there is no wrong way to create fajitas, as long as fresh ingredients are used. This vegetarian version is loaded with the freshest farmers market ingredients. I am sure that it's destined to become a conversation piece at your dinner table, too!

8 flour tortillas
1 Tablespoon olive oil
2 medium zucchini, julienned
2 carrots, peeled and julienned
1 Vidalia onion, sliced thin
1 red pepper, julienned
½ pound mushrooms, sliced
Juice of ½ lime
¼ cup chopped fresh cilantro
1 (16-ounce) can black beans, rinsed and drained
½ cup vegetable stock
½ teaspoon cumin
1 teaspoon hot sauce
1 bay leaf
½ teaspoon garlic powder
Pepper to taste

Accompaniments:
    ½ avocado, cubed
    4 ounces shredded Monterey Jack or
        cheddar cheese
    Sour cream
    Salsa
    2 tomatoes, seeded and chopped

Preheat oven to 350 degrees. Wrap tortillas in aluminum foil and set aside. In large, non-stick skillet, heat olive oil over medium-high heat. When oil is hot but not smoking, add onions and peppers and sauté for 2 minutes. Add zucchini and carrots and sauté until slightly tender, 4-5 minutes. Add mushrooms and sauté, tossing frequently with other vegetables. Season with salt and pepper, squeeze fresh lime over vegetables and turn heat to low. Meanwhile, in medium sauce pan, heat rinsed and drained black beans over medium heat. Add vegetable stock and bring just to boil. Add cumin, bay leaf and hot sauce and stir to combine. Reduce heat to low and simmer 10 minutes. Warm foil-wrapped tortillas in oven for 10 minutes. Serve tortillas, vegetables, bean filling and accompaniments at once, and watch the fun begin!

Serves 4.

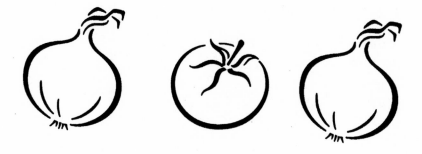

CROSS CREEK AJIACO

Ajiaco (a-hi-a-ko) is a delicious Colombian soup loaded with chicken, corn, cilantro and a variety of potatoes, then garnished with avocado and capers. This soup is traditional throughout Latin America and each country has its own special creation. My version comes from my cousin Suzanne and her husband John, who collected this recipe while living in South America. Now, each time we visit their charming farmhouse and orange grove in Cross Creek, Florida, we are welcomed with a steaming bowl of Ajiaco.

2 (15-ounce) cans chicken broth, preferably low-sodium

8 cups of water (more, if needed)

1 pound boneless, skinless chicken breasts

1 large yellow onion, coarsely chopped, with ends reserved

2 celery stalks, sliced, with ends reserved

1 large bunch fresh cilantro, rinsed clean and coarsely chopped, with ends reserved

2 ears fresh corn, husked and cut into 2- to 3-inch pieces

2 cups Yukon gold potatoes, peeled and cut into 2-inch pieces

2 cups fingerling potatoes, peeled and cut into 2-inch pieces

2 cups red skin potatoes, peeled and cut into 2-inch pieces

2 medium carrots, peeled and sliced

1 avocado, peeled and cubed

Capers

Sour cream

In large saucepan, combine chicken broth with water, reserved cilantro, onion and celery ends and chicken. Bring liquid to boil and simmer chicken until cooked through, about 15 minutes. Remove chicken and let cool on plate. Remove onion, celery and cilantro stems. You should now have a flavorful stock. Add chopped potatoes, carrots, onion and celery and simmer, uncovered, 30 minutes until potatoes are just tender. Meanwhile, shred cooked chicken into bite-size pieces. Add corn, chicken and cilantro and simmer 5 minutes until all flavors are blended. Season with salt and pepper. Serve in bowls and garnish with avocado, capers and a dollop of sour cream.

Serves 6.

Quick Tip: If you can't find fingerling potatoes, use russet potatoes.

PENNE PRIMAVERA WITH FETA

This is one of my weeknight standby recipes, for times when I just can't deal with anything too complicated. True to its primavera roots, this is a wholesome and tasty pasta dish full of colorful vegetables. If there are any leftovers, they will make a great lunch!

1 clove garlic, minced
2 teaspoons olive oil
4 scallions, sliced
8-10 mushrooms, sliced
1 red bell pepper, coarsely chopped
1 medium zucchini, julienned
¾ pound asparagus, cut into 2-inch pieces
¼ cup white wine,
¼ cup vegetable broth
8-10 cherry tomatoes, halved
1/3 cup fresh Italian parsley, chopped
1/3 cup fresh basil, chopped
4 ounces feta cheese, crumbled
1 pound penne pasta, cooked al dente and drained

Heat olive oil in large, non-stick skillet over medium heat. When oil is warm, add garlic and scallions. Stir until just soft and fragrant, about 2 minutes. Add mushrooms and red pepper and sauté 3 minutes. Add white wine and broth and bring to simmer. Add zucchini and asparagus and simmer over medium-low heat for 6-8 minutes (or until asparagus is crisply tender). Meanwhile, cook pasta according to directions for al dente. Add parsley, basil and cherry tomatoes to vegetable mixture and continue simmering for 3-4 minutes. Remove from heat. Drain pasta and toss with vegetables and feta cheese.

Serves 4.

ASIAN STIR-FRY PASTA

Low in fat but rich with flavor, this pasta dish is loaded with crisp vegetables and seasoned with an exotic dressing. This recipe's best feature, however, is its simplicity. It makes a perfect casual weeknight dinner and is a great antidote for a long, hectic day.

2 teaspoons peanut oil
1 clove garlic, minced
4 scallions, sliced
1 Tablespoon fresh ginger, finely minced
½ cup pea pods or sugar snap peas, trimmed
½ cup broccoli, chopped into florets
½ cup asparagus, chopped into 1-inch pieces
1 red pepper, sliced julienne
½ cup mushrooms, sliced
¼ cup water chestnuts
2 carrots, peeled, sliced and julienned
1 Tablespoon soy sauce
1/3 cup plus 1 Tablespoon Asian sesame dressing
½ pound linguine or fettuccine
2 Tablespoons roasted peanuts, coarsely chopped
¼ cup fresh cilantro, chopped

For Sesame Vinaigrette:
½ teaspoon sugar
2 Tablespoons soy sauce
3 Tablespoons rice vinegar
Juice of one lime
1 teaspoon hot sauce or Asian chili sauce
2 Tablespoons honey
1 garlic clove, minced
1 Tablespoon hoisin sauce*
1 Tablespoon sesame oil
2 Tablespoons peanut oil
1 Tablespoon scallion, minced

    1 Tablespoon cilantro, minced

    1 Tablespoon fresh ginger, minced

    2 teaspoons sesame seeds, toasted and cooled (optional)

*Available at most grocery stores, gourmet markets or Asian markets.

Combine sugar, soy sauce, vinegar, lime juice, hot sauce, honey, garlic and hoison sauce in medium bowl and whisk together. Add oils slowly and whisk vigorously. Add scallion, cilantro, ginger and sesame seeds and whisk again. Stores easily in refrigerator for up to 2 weeks.

Heat peanut oil in wok and stir-fry garlic, scallions and fresh ginger for 30 seconds. Add vegetables, soy sauce and 1 Tablespoon Asian dressing. Stir-fry vegetables until crisply tender or to desired texture. Meanwhile, in large pot, cook pasta al dente, according to package instructions. Drain pasta in colander and place in large bowl or wok with heat turned off. Toss with vegetables and remaining dressing. Serve onto plates and sprinkle with roasted peanuts and cilantro.

    Serves 2-4.

Variations: You can use any selection of your favorite vegetables. Try bok choy, spinach, bean sprouts or zucchini for an even wider range of flavors.

PLUM TOMATO PASTA

Here is my favorite fresh tomato sauce which uses the lively flavor of balsamic vinegar to enrich the sweetness of tomatoes and reduce their acidity. I like to use capellini for this recipe, which is traditional for this type of preparation. Tube pastas such as penne or rigatoni also work well, because they help to "cup" this delicious sauce.

> 1½ pounds fresh plum tomatoes, peeled, seeded and
>   coarsely chopped
> 1 Tablespoon olive oil
> 1 garlic clove, minced
> 5 large green olives, sliced
> 3 Tablespoons balsamic vinegar
> ¼ cup fresh basil, chopped
> 2 Tablespoons fresh parsley, chopped
> 12 ounces angel hair pasta or spaghettini
> ¼ cup Parmesan cheese, grated

In large skillet, heat olive oil and garlic over medium-low heat and cook until garlic is translucent. Increase heat to medium and add tomatoes. Simmer for 12-15 minutes. Add vinegar and olives and simmer for 5 minutes. Add basil and parsley and simmer over low heat for another 5-10 minutes. Meanwhile, cook pasta according to directions. Drain pasta. Spoon sauce over hot pasta and sprinkle with fresh Parmesan cheese.

Serves 2-4.

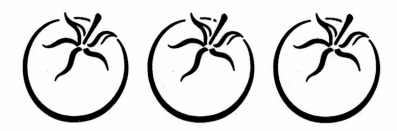

MEDITERRANEAN PENNE PASTA

This healthful and satisfying pasta is created with ingredients you can keep on hand in your freezer or pantry, plus the best vine-ripened tomatoes you can find. The delicious union of spinach, tomatoes, feta and pine nuts will bring a Mediterranean flair to your dinner table and a new favorite to your family.

16 ounces penne pasta
1 garlic clove, minced
2 Tablespoons olive oil
1 (10-ounce) package frozen, chopped spinach, thawed
    and drained well
2 large vine-ripened tomatoes, seeded and chopped
1 cup mushrooms, sliced
4 ounces crumbled feta cheese
¼ cup toasted pine nuts
Black pepper to taste

In non-stick skillet, heat 1 Tablespoon oil and garlic over medium heat until fragrant. Add mushrooms and sauté until tender. Add spinach and tomatoes and sauté until tomatoes are just tender. Meanwhile, cook pasta al dente. Season with pepper and keep sauce warm. Drain pasta. Toss with remaining olive oil and then with spinach and tomato mixture. Drizzle with more olive oil (1 Tablespoon at most), if needed. Add feta cheese and toss again. Serve in pasta dish and sprinkle with pine nuts.

Serves 4.

Quick Tip: If you prefer, use one 12-ounce bag of fresh spinach. Make sure to buy spinach that has already been cleaned.

PASTA WITH CHICKEN, FENNEL
AND
SUN-DRIED TOMATOES

It's hard to go wrong when creating pasta dishes. Here is a fantastic blend of wholesome ingredients, resulting in a substantial main course. Fennel is a vegetable often used in Greek and Mediterranean cooking. Rich in vitamin A, it becomes sweeter when cooked, releasing a mild anise flavor. Here, fennel, sun-dried tomatoes and carrots lend their sweet aroma to chicken and penne. Filled with a warm and inviting character, this pasta dish redefines comfort food.

12 ounces penne pasta
2 Tablespoons olive oil
½ teaspoon fennel seeds
½ teaspoon crushed red pepper
½ cup Vidalia onion, chopped
1 whole boneless, skinless chicken breast (8-10 ounces),
    rimmed and cut into small strips
1 cup white button mushrooms, sliced
1 fennel bulb, trimmed and cut crosswise into strips
2 carrots, peeled and julienned
1/3 cup sun-dried tomatoes (without oil), soaked in hot
    water to cover for 5 minutes, and then chopped
½ cup vegetable or chicken broth
¼ cup fresh basil, chopped
2 ounces freshly grated Asiago cheese

In large skillet, heat olive oil over medium-high heat until warm. Add fennel seeds, red pepper and onion and sauté until onion is just softened, about 4 minutes. Add chicken and sauté until cooked through and no longer pink. Transfer chicken to plate with slotted spoon and keep warm. Add mushrooms, fennel bulb and carrots to pan and sauté until just lightly golden. Add broth and simmer, about 5 minutes. Return chicken to skillet and add sun-dried tomatoes. Toss well. Meanwhile, cook pasta al dente. Drain pasta and combine with sauce. Toss with fresh basil and Asiago cheese and serve.

Serves 2-4.

Quick Tip: If you have never used fresh fennel, don't be intimidated. It is a delicious vegetable and fairly easy to find in your local market. Choose white, round stalks with leaves, if possible. To prepare fennel, trim off end that looks like a celery stalk and discard. Slice fennel bulb as thin as possible. Immerse cut fennel in cold water to clean. Discard feather leaves and narrow stalks. Wrap fennel in plastic and keep in refrigerator.

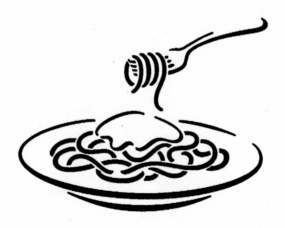

ALFRESCO TOMATO ARUGULA PASTA

This delicious dish of hot pasta tossed with a cool tomato sauce reminds me of alfresco dining, sipping a cool drink at an outdoor cafe under a warm, inviting sun. Applying the instant heat of the pasta to the tomatoes brings out their full flavor. Crisp arugula adds a peppery bite, creating a sensational union of ingredients. Choose plump, ripe plum tomatoes or flavor-packed, vine-ripened tomatoes for best results.

1 pound fettuccine
1½ pounds fresh plum tomatoes, seeded and coarsely
    chopped
1 Tablespoon extra-virgin olive oil
1 Tablespoon lemon juice
2 Tablespoons balsamic vinegar
½ cup fresh basil, chopped
3 Tablespoons fresh flat leaf parsley, chopped
6 large green olives, sliced
1 small bunch of arugula, washed, trimmed and coarsely
    chopped
Fresh ground pepper to taste
2 ounces feta cheese, crumbled (optional)

In large bowl, combine tomatoes, olive oil, lemon juice, balsamic vinegar, basil, parsley and olives. Season with pepper. Cover and chill for 30 minutes. Bring large pot of water to boil and cook fettuccine according to al dente instructions. Toss hot pasta with cold tomato mixture, sprinkle with feta cheese and serve.

Serves 4.

Variation: For a more colorful dish substitute half of the tomatoes with ripe yellow tomatoes.

LIGHT-HEAVYWEIGHT CHAMPION PASTA

My godfather, Willie Pastrano, was a world champion light-heavyweight boxer. He and his wife Faye were renowned cooks who grew up in Miami, so although this is a classic Italian creation, it certainly has strong Florida roots. This pasta entree was inspired by her recipe, which was handed down through our family. The pork tenderloin is an uncommon addition, which adds lean and mean satisfaction for a powerful pasta meal.

2 Tablespoons olive oil
1-pound pork tenderloin, cut into ¾-inch slices
3 cloves garlic, blanched and sliced
2½ pounds fresh plum tomatoes, peeled, seeded and
coarsely chopped
2 Tablespoons fresh parsley
1 teaspoon dried oregano
2 Tablespoons tomato paste
½ cup water
¼ cup dry red wine
Salt and pepper to taste
1 pound linguine or fettuccine
Freshly grated Parmesan cheese (optional)

In large skillet, heat olive oil over medium-high heat and sauté tenderloin slices 5-7 minutes on both sides. Remove pork from skillet. Drain olive oil from pan. In same skillet, over medium heat, add tomatoes and garlic and bring to simmer. Simmer over low heat about 20 minutes. Add parsley, oregano, tomato paste, ½ cup of water and red wine. Stir until smooth. Add tenderloin to sauce and simmer 5-10 minutes longer. Season with salt and pepper to taste. Meanwhile, cook pasta, al dente, according to package instructions. Serve pasta with sauce. Sprinkle with Parmesan.

Serves 4-6.

Quick Tip: *To peel and seed tomatoes, use small, sharp knife to make an "X" in tip of tomato opposite stem. Bring pot of water to boil and place tomatoes in pot. Boil for 2 minutes, drain tomatoes in colander and rinse with cold water to cool. If peeling does not easily slip off, remove stubborn areas with small, sharp knife. To seed tomatoes, cut in half crosswise and gently squeeze or use an index finger to scoop seeds out.*

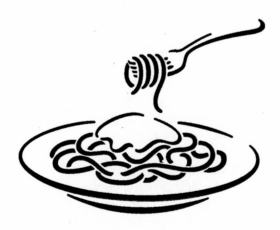

RED WINE-INFUSED BEEF KABOBS

The key to successful kabobs is using a great marinade and fresh vegetables to complement a great cut of beef. Kabobs are the quintessential backyard barbecue entree. So the really essential ingredients are a crisp, cool breeze and a fabulous Florida sunset!

For marinade:
½ cup peanut oil
¼ cup soy sauce
2 Tablespoons Worcestershire sauce
2 Tablespoons dry mustard
1 Tablespoon coarse salt
1 Tablespoon fresh ground pepper
1 cup red wine
3 Tablespoons fresh parsley, chopped
1/3 cup fresh lemon juice

For kabobs:
1-pound beef tenderloin or flank steak cut into 2-inch pieces
2 red bell peppers, seeded and cut into 8 pieces each
1 red onion, quartered and separated into 8 pieces
2 Portabello mushrooms sliced into ½-inch thick pieces
8 cherry tomatoes (or more)

Prepare marinade by whisking all ingredients in bowl. Reserve about 1/3 cup marinade and set aside. Marinate beef and vegetables for 2-4 hours. Thread pieces onto skewers, alternating beef, pepper, mushroom, onion and tomatoes. Grill over high heat to preferred temperature, 6-7 minutes per side for medium.

Serves 4.

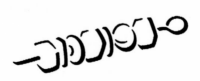

BOURBON BALSAMIC BARBECUE PORK TENDERLOIN

Pork tenderloin has certainly become a favorite entrée of many chefs. It is lean, tender, versatile and delicious. This recipe is most often requested by my friends and family, which is great, because it is a cinch to make. It has a tangy, unforgettable barbecue flavor laced with a hint of bourbon.

1½-pound pork tenderloin
Coarse salt
Fresh cracked black pepper
3 Tablespoons bourbon
2 Tablespoons light brown sugar
2 Tablespoons balsamic vinegar
2 Tablespoons fresh ginger, grated
3 Tablespoons Dijon mustard
3 Tablespoons chili sauce
1 teaspoon hot sauce

Rinse tenderloin, pat dry and sprinkle with salt and pepper. Combine next 7 ingredients in medium sauce pan and bring to boil. Stir to dissolve sugar and remove from heat. Prepare grill. Grill tenderloin over medium heat, about 6 minutes per side (or to your preference), basting frequently with sauce. Remove tenderloin from grill. (It should still be slightly pink in center.) Meat will continue to cook after you remove it from heat. Let sit for 10 minutes, then slice into ½-inch pieces and serve.

Serves 4.

Quick Tip: According to my bourbon experts, authentic bourbon comes only from Kentucky. If you don't have the real thing on hand, however, Jack Daniel's is an acceptable substitute.

SKILLET-SEARED LAMB CHOPS
WITH
LEMON, ARTICHOKES AND DILL

Compact and juicy, lamb chops have a wonderful, earthy flavor. This upscale main course is terrific as a special dinner for two. Sautéing lamb chops will seal in their flavor, and the artichokes, lemon and dill will add a pleasing, distinctive zest.

> 2 Tablespoons olive oil
> Four 1-inch thick lamb loin chops
> 1 clove garlic, minced
> 8 artichoke hearts, quartered
> ¼ cup white wine
> Juice of one lemon
> 1 Tablespoon fresh dill, chopped, or 1 teaspoon dried
>   dill
> Salt and pepper to taste
> 1 lemon for garnish, sliced thin

In non-stick skillet, heat 1 Tablespoon olive oil over medium-high heat. Add lamb chops and sauté until done to your preference, 3-4 minutes per side for medium-rare or 4-5 minutes per side for medium. Remove from heat and set aside, keeping covered and warm. Add remaining Tablespoon olive oil to skillet. Add artichoke hearts, wine, lemon and dill and simmer 3-4 minutes over low heat, until wine is reduced and sauce is glazed. Return lamb chops to pan and coat with sauce. Season with salt and pepper. Garnish with lemon slices and serve.

Serves 2.

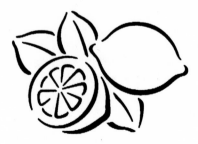

CLASSIC VEAL PICCATA

Some recipes never lose their charm. I grew up with this classic main course, which was one of my mother's signature dishes. Veal is an elegant, lean and protein-rich entree. Here, a delicate blend of lemon, wine and capers brings out its full, tender flavor.

½ pound veal medallions
1 Tablespoon olive oil
2 Tablespoons butter
1/3 cup fresh lemon juice
¼ cup white wine
1 Tablespoon capers
2 Tablespoons fresh parsley
Salt and pepper to taste
1 lemon sliced into ¼-inch pieces

Rinse veal medallions, pat dry and sprinkle with salt and pepper. In medium skillet, heat olive oil over medium heat and sauté veal medallions until browned, about 4 minutes per side. Remove veal and keep warm. Add butter, lemon juice, white wine and capers and simmer until reduced by half, about 6 minutes. Add cornstarch and water mixture and simmer another 2 minutes until sauce is glazed. Add parsley and season with salt and pepper to taste. Pour sauce over veal and garnish with lemon slices.

Serves 2.

Speaking of Lemons...Four different varieties of lemons grow in Florida: the Eureka, Lisbon, Ponderosa and Meyer.

Eureka lemon has a smooth, attractive, lemon-yellow skin. This lemon does not have a pronounced tip like many others. It has a few seeds, is high in acid, good for juice and would work well with this recipe.

Ponderosa lemon is not a true lemon, and it is certainly not an attractive fruit. Larger and pear-shaped, it has a thick, bumpy rind and makes a good marmalade or preserve.

Meyer lemon is highly sought after by today's chefs for its high juice content and excellent flavor. These lemons are juicy and less acidic than most.

Lisbon lemon is probably the most popular lemon. It has the familiar lemon shape, a pronounced tip, and a versatile flavor, and it's good for most recipes.

Chapter 5

Killer Sweet-Tooth Treats

Tropical Fruit Pizza
Carmelized Peaches
Flan de la Finca
Beehive Coconut Pie
Coconut Snowballs with Dark Chocolate Sauce
Banana Coconut Rum Cake
Creamsicle Chiffon Pie
Frozen Lime Pie
Stargazers

TROPICAL FRUIT PIZZA

This dessert is ideal for a party. If you have any helping hands around the house, it can be ready in snap. It's a great creative outlet for kids or guests, and everyone will devour the results. Using fresh fruits in season, you can make this dessert any time of year!

For crust:
- ½ cup butter, melted
- ¼ cup oatmeal
- ¼ cup chopped pecans
- 1 cup graham cracker crumbs

For topping:
- 1 pint vanilla yogurt
- ¼ cup lemon juice
- 1 (14-ounce) can regular or low-fat sweetened condensed milk
- 1 teaspoon vanilla

Mixture of tropical fruits including:
- 1 fresh papaya, peeled and sliced
- 1 fresh pineapple, cored, peeled and cut into wedges
- 1 pint fresh strawberries, sliced
- 2 fresh peaches, sliced
- 3 fresh kiwi, sliced
- 2 fresh bananas, sliced
- 1 cup raspberries
- 1 cup blueberries

Preheat oven to 375 degrees. In medium mixing bowl, mix crust ingredients together to form a crumbly dough. Press into 12-inch round, ungreased pizza pan or tart pan. Bake 11-13 minutes or until golden. Cool completely. Mix yogurt, lemon juice, condensed milk and vanilla. Chill until slightly firm, about 1 hour. Spread topping over cooled crust and decorate with fruit. Chill tart about 1 hour prior to serving. Cut into slices and serve.

Serves 6-8.

> *Quick Tip: Brush fruit with 1 Tablespoon lemon juice mixed with 1 teaspoon honey after assembling the pizza. This will prevent fruit from browning and give it a fresh presentation.*

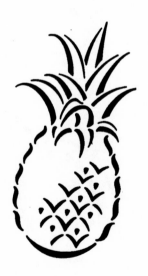

CARMELIZED PEACHES

Fresh, juicy peaches are the ultimate summer indulgence. Although Florida is not known for peach production, peaches from our Georgia neighbors make their way each season to our best markets. This sauce takes advantage of their exquisite sweetness, creating a richly flavored, syrupy dessert.

  3 ripe peaches, peeled and sliced
  1 Tablespoon butter
  3 Tablespoons light brown sugar
  3 Tablespoons fresh-squeezed orange juice
  2 Tablespoons Grand Marnier liqueur
  1 pint vanilla ice cream or frozen yogurt

In non-stick skillet, melt butter over medium heat. Add butter, brown sugar, orange juice and liqueur and bring to simmer, stirring constantly to avoid burning. Add peaches and stir to coat with caramel. Simmer over low heat until peaches are softened. Serve over vanilla ice cream or frozen yogurt.

Serves 4.

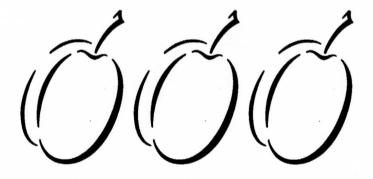

FLAN DE LA FINCA

This beloved custard dessert is a Spanish-inspired version created by my Aunt Carol, who owns an avocado farm in Malaga. "Finca" means farm in Spanish, so it's only natural that this creation would have an authentic, home-style quality. When she is in Malaga, Carol loves to entertain friends, and this is one of her mainstay desserts.

1 cup sugar
1 quart milk
1 Tablespoon butter
½ cup sugar
½ teaspoon salt
1 cup dried bread cubes (optional)
8 eggs, beaten
1 Tablespoon dark rum or vanilla

Preheat oven to 350 degrees. In medium saucepan, bring 1 cup sugar to boil over medium-low heat until it caramelizes and just begins to smoke. Remove from heat immediately and pour caramel into custard mold. In large saucepan over medium heat, combine milk, salt, butter and ½ cup sugar. Let sugar dissolve, then scald milk, heating until small bubbles appear on outside edge of mixture. Remove from heat. Add beaten eggs and 1 Tablespoon dark rum or vanilla. Mix and pour into mold. Place mold into baking pan or bottom of broiler pan with about 1" of water in bottom. Bake in oven for 1 hour or until inserted knife comes out clean. If using bread cubes, add to mixture halfway through cooking process. When cool, loosen with knife and invert onto serving plate.

Serves 8.

Variation: Flan is an outstanding dessert on its own but if you want to add a tropical theme, serve it with sliced mango or strawberries, which will intensify the caramel flavor.

BEEHIVE COCONUT PIE

This is an authentic island coconut pie recipe from our friends Bo and Joyce, who have spent many summers on their boat in the Bahamas, fishing, diving and sweet-talking native bakers into revealing their secret ingredients. Sinfully rich with coconut flavor, this pie is worth every calorie you consume!

3 eggs
1 teaspoon vanilla
1 Tablespoon flour
1½ cups shredded sweetened coconut
½ cup buttermilk
6 Tablespoons butter, softened
1 prepared, uncooked pie crust
½ teaspoon nutmeg (optional)

Preheat oven to 350 degrees. Beat together eggs and vanilla. Add flour, coconut, buttermilk and butter and beat until smooth. Pour mixture into uncooked pie crust, sprinkle top with nutmeg and bake 1 hour. During last 20 minutes, cover top of pie with aluminum foil to prevent burning. Let cool completely and serve.

Serves 6-8.

> *Quick Tip: Many cooks are intimidated at the thought of making fresh pie crust, but it is not difficult and the results are worth the effort. I prefer flaky butter crust for most of my pies: In food processor, combine 2 cups all-purpose flour with 2 sticks cold unsalted butter, cut into ½-inch cubes. Process until mixture resembles oatmeal. While processing, add 1/3 cup water in stream until dough forms ball. Remove dough from processor and divide it into three equal parts. Shape each part into a disc and wrap with plastic wrap. Chill 30 minutes. Remove one disc from refrigerator and roll it into 11-inch circle. Use additional flour as needed to keep rolling pin from sticking. Place pie crust into ungreased pie pan and chill until needed.*

COCONUT SNOWBALLS
WITH
DARK CHOCOLATE SAUCE

This is one of those "back-up" dessert recipes that makes you look as if you have worked hard in the kitchen. If you have these ingredients on hand, there is nothing to the preparation. Be inventive with your presentation: Serve this dessert in a chilled martini glass with a sprig of mint or on a decorative plate with sauce drizzled around edges.

2 cups shredded sweetened coconut
1 quart chocolate or vanilla frozen yogurt or ice cream
1/3 cup brewed coffee
½ cup packed brown sugar
½ cup unsweetened Dutch process cocoa
3 Tablespoons unsalted butter, cut into pieces
1 teaspoon vanilla
2 Tablespoons coconut rum or liqueur

Preheat oven to 325 degrees. Spread coconut on baking sheet and toast in oven for about 10 minutes. Do not burn. Cool coconut. Using ice cream scoop, spoon out round ice cream balls and roll one at a time in toasted coconut until coated, pressing coconut into ice cream with your fingers if necessary. Place ice cream balls in large, air-tight container and freeze until ready to serve. Meanwhile, in heavy saucepan, heat coffee with brown sugar over medium-high heat, whisking until sugar is dissolved. Add cocoa powder and salt, whisking until smooth. Add butter, vanilla and coconut rum and whisk until butter is melted and sauce is smooth. Keep sauce warm. To serve, place 2 Tablespoons sauce on plate or in serving dish and top with coconut snowballs.

Serves 6.

> *Quick Tip: To prevent shredded coconut from burning while toasting, check on it often and stir occasionally. Remember, oven temperatures vary and coconut will burn in seconds.*

BANANA COCONUT RUM CAKE

My mother-in-law made traditional coconut cakes for my husband's birthday every year. I never thought I could live up to the challenge of duplicating her signature dessert. But this moist, sweet and light cake just might be his new favorite—although he won't admit it!

For cake:
> 3 medium bananas, mashed
> 1/3 cup coconut rum
> 2 cups cake flour
> ½ teaspoon salt
> ¾ teaspoon baking soda
> ½ teaspoon baking powder
> 1 cup sugar
> ½ cup brown sugar
> ½ cup butter, softened
> 2 teaspoons vanilla
> 2 eggs
> ¼ cup buttermilk
> 1 cup shredded sweetened coconut

For glaze:
> 2 Tablespoons melted butter
> 2 Tablespoons water
> ½ cup sugar
> ¼ cup coconut rum

For whipped cream frosting:
> 1 cup whipped cream
> 3 Tablespoons sugar
> ¼ cup shredded sweetened coconut, lightly toasted

Preheat oven to 350. Grease two 9-inch cake pans and dust with flour. Mash
. bananas with 2 Tablespoons coconut rum and soak for 15 minutes. Sift cake
flour, salt, soda and baking powder separately. In large bowl, beat butter and
sugars until fluffy. Add eggs, vanilla and buttermilk; beat until well blended.
Add sifted ingredients to butter mixture, alternating with mashed bananas and
beating in two segments. Beat in coconut, pour batter into cake pans and bake
30-35 minutes. Remove from oven and cool to room temperature. Meanwhile,
melt butter with sugar and water over medium heat. Stir to dissolve sugar, boil 5
minutes, remove from heat and add rum. Remove cooled cake from pans. Poke
several holes in layers with toothpick. Brush layers with rum mixture (glaze),
using all or part. Combine whipping cream with sugar. Beat on high until stiff,
but not dry. Frost cake with whipped cream and sprinkle top with toasted
coconut.

Serves 8-10.

CREAMSICLE CHIFFON PIE

This sinfully delicious dessert captures that unforgettable creamy orange Popsicle taste we all craved as kids. I came up with this recipe after a neighbor dropped off a bushel of calamondins. The tart acidity of this tangerine and kumquat relative lends itself perfectly to a fluffy and sweet chiffon pie. If you can't find calamondins, add the juice of a lemon to freshly squeezed orange juice.

For crust:
  1 cup graham cracker crumbs
  ½ cup sweetened coconut, grated
  ¼ cup butter, melted

For pie:
  3 eggs, separated
  1 (14-ounce) can sweetened condensed milk
  2/3 cup calamondin juice
  2 Tablespoons fresh orange zest

For topping:
  ½ cup heavy cream
  3 Tablespoons sugar

Preheat oven to 350 degrees. Butter 9-inch pie dish. In medium bowl, combine graham cracker crumbs, coconut and melted butter and toss well. Pour crumb mixture into pie dish and press firmly and evenly until crust is formed. Bake in oven for 8-10 minutes or until golden. In large bowl, beat egg yolks and zest on high speed until fluffy and lemon-colored, about 4 minutes. Add condensed milk and beat until thick and smooth, about 3 minutes. Add calamondin or tart orange juice in stream while mixer is on low, mixing until blended. In medium bowl, beat egg whites until stiff. Fold egg whites into egg yolk mixture and pour into crust. Bake in oven for 20-25 minutes or until lightly golden on top. Remove from oven and cool. Refrigerate for 1 hour. In medium bowl, combine cream and sugar and beat until cream holds firm peaks. Top pie with whipped cream to decorate or spread evenly on top, and serve.

Serves 6-8.

FROZEN LIME PIE

Key lime pie is as much a tradition in Florida as clam chowder is in New England. Handed down to me by my mother-in-law, Carmer, this frozen lime pie recipe has a refreshing twist that rivals any other version. We use Persian limes, which are available all year round and provide a greater volume of juice than other varieties. It's a perfect ending to any meal and a tradition worth keeping.

For crust:
   1¼ cup graham cracker crumbs
   ¼ cup butter, melted
   ½ cup shredded sweetened coconut

For filling:
   4 eggs, separated
   ½ cup lime juice (preferably Persian lime)
   1 can sweetened condensed milk
   Pinch of salt
   Grated rind of 1 lime

Preheat oven to 350 degrees. Butter 9-inch pie pan or spray with non-stick cooking spray. In medium bowl, combine one cup graham cracker crumbs, melted butter and coconut and mix until well blended. Pour crumbs into pie pan, pressing firmly and evenly to form crust. Bake in oven for 8-10 minutes or until golden. In large bowl, beat egg yolks until pale. Add sweetened condensed milk, lime juice and salt and mix until smooth. In medium bowl, mix egg whites until stiff. Fold egg whites into egg yolk mixture and fold in lime peel. Pour into crust. Sprinkle top with remaining graham cracker crumbs and freeze 6-8 hours.

Serves 8-10.

Limes Galore: *Florida grows plenty of limes and is known commercially for 2 of its varieties, Key lime and Persian lime. Key limes produce a highly acidic juice and seedy fruit. They are known to grow wild and are found throughout South Florida and along some coastlines. They mature in summer, but some fruit can be found year-round. Persian limes are the most commercially popular lime. Available all year round, they are a seedless, acidic fruit. These limes are utilized extensively in cooking, as well as in drinks, dressings, marinades, sauces and other preparations.*

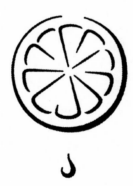

STARGAZERS

In the Bahamas, we call this drink a Nasty Royale. It's a great combination of an after-dinner drink and a rich chocolate dessert, sipped warm out of a cup. This is about as elaborate as a dessert menu gets in the Bahamas after a day of fishing and diving. After a fabulous meal, we have just enough energy to mix these delicious concoctions, sit on the deck and gaze at the stars.

> 1 can International Foods Suisse Mocha coffee mix
> 36 ounces hot water
> ¾ cup Nassau Royale liqueur
> 1 cup heavy whipping cream
> 1 teaspoon vanilla

Mix 2 heaping Tablespoons of Suisse Mocha mix to each 6 ounces of hot water and stir until well blended. Add 2 ounces of Nassau Royale liqueur and stir again. Whip cream with vanilla until it holds stiff peaks. Serve whipped cream on top of each coffee drink.

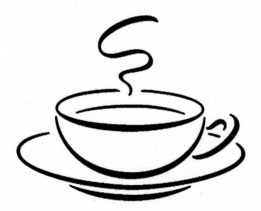

Chapter 6:

Making Life Easier

For those of us who love it, cooking is a nurturing and creative process. I've always believed the key to gaining true pleasure from this process is having the ability to create a meal on the spur of the moment. In order to accomplish this, you should have essential ingredients stocked in your pantry, as well as a few basic kitchen tools.

As I've mentioned, the recipes in Florida's Backyard offer a relaxed, simple style of cooking. You don't have to be an expertly trained chef with full access to every piece of culinary equipment to be successful in the kitchen. Those of us who are resourceful with a few tools can have as much fun as those fortunate cooks with a completely outfitted kitchen. My advice is to keep it simple, experiment, have fun, and to use your senses and your good sense to taste and enjoy!

Having said that, I offer you some guidelines to make using this book easier and to improve your overall knowledge of cooking with fresh, Florida ingredients.

Common Ingredients Used in *Florida's Backyard* Recipes

★ *Olive Oil* Olive oil is the cooking fat I prefer, and I use extra virgin oil because of its rich flavor. You don't need an expensive olive oil, especially for sautéing foods, when it's actually better to use a less expensive pure olive oil. And don't use the "light" olive oil thinking it contains less fat. Actually, it's just a lower grade, diluted olive oil that lacks flavor. Do use a high-grade extra virgin oil for salad dressings and sauces, however. I prefer Spanish olive oils for their aroma and fruity flavor. I specifically recommend Virgin Gold, which is available through Iberian Products USA, 1-610-587-5470.

★ *Butter* When butter is called for, use the sweet, unsalted variety.

★ *Hot Sauces* My personal taste is to use hot sauces often in my recipes. I like Tiger Sauce, because it has a touch of corn syrup, which balances its spicy pepper flavor. Cholula, a Mexican hot sauce is also a good brand. There are so many varieties of hot sauces at the markets, you may have to try a few to find the brand you like best. My recipes are going to taste best with a traditional hot pepper sauce, so if you cannot find Tiger Sauce, I recommend Tabasco Sauce, Louisiana Hot Sauce or a Caribbean-style hot sauce. If you don't like spicy foods, you can always season to taste, or omit the sauce.

★ *Juices and Nectars* I lighten many of my recipes with juices and nectars. I use only freshly squeezed citrus juices. In a pinch, you can use prepared orange juice, but never use bottled lemon or lime juice because the flavor is non-existent in cooking. I often use nectars for their dense body and full flavor. You can find canned nectars, such as papaya, mango, passion fruit or guava in the canned fruit juice section of most markets or at a good health food store.

★ *Fresh Herbs* I prefer fresh herbs to dried ones. If you can't find a specific herb, you have two choices: (a) Substitute an available fresh herb, or (b) Use the dried version. If you substitute a fresh herb, the taste will be slightly altered, but if you use the proper substitution, the flavor will be retained. For example:

- Basil, mint, and parsley can be used interchangeably in most recipes and are compatible with each other. They substitute well for each other in most salsa, sauces, and soups.
- Thyme, parsley, oregano, and basil can be used interchangeably in pasta dishes. Mint, oregano, and rosemary are good partners with certain meats, such as lamb.
- If you're preparing seafood and are low on herbs, thyme is always a good standby, because its flavor is compatible with virtually any seafood.
- Thyme, rosemary, mint, and parsley are excellent flavor enhancers for potatoes and vegetables.
- Certain herbs have such distinctive flavors that it's difficult to substitute for them. For example:

  - Dill has a unique character and is difficult to replace, although dried dill holds its flavor well and is a good alternative to fresh.
  - Tarragon's peppery-anise flavor is also tricky to replace, but you may use basil on some occasions.
  - Sage, used most often in poultry dishes, meats, and winter vegetables, also has a unique character, but you can use the dried version with success.
  - Because Marjoram has a minty flavor, it can stand in for mint, or vice-versa.

- Cilantro, with its pungent citrusy aroma, is an herb with a strong personality, so it's difficult to replace in salsa or sauces. Mint or basil are the best alternatives. Remember, if you plan to use the dried version of any herb in a recipe, be sure it's fresh; dried herbs should be replaced yearly, or even every six months.

★ *Spices* Unlike dried herbs, spices such as peppercorns, cumin, nutmeg, cinnamon, and others will keep for up to two years and will retain their best flavor when frozen. They release a more pungent flavor if you buy them whole and grind them with a mortar and pestle or in a spice grinder. This technique works particularly well with black or white peppercorns, which I use often in my recipes.

★ *Zest* "Zest" refers to the outer peel of citrus fruit, which should be free of the bitter white pith. To obtain zest, it's best to use a kitchen tool known as a "zester," a fine grater or a vegetable peeler.

★ *Kosher Salt* Using kosher salt in place of standard table salt is an invaluable way to season foods, because it possesses a clean taste and a coarse texture. Also, kosher salt has no additives, so it's milder in flavor and more pure than traditional table salt. It also does an excellent job of tenderizing meats and bringing out the flavor in vegetables, vinaigrettes, and sauces. Sea salt has a clean taste also, and can be used if kosher salt is unavailable. Remember that regular table salt has the strongest, harshest flavor. As a general rule when using any salt, always season to taste.

★ *Nuts and Seeds* I use a variety of nuts and seeds throughout my recipes to add flavor, nutrition, and texture, and generally recommend they are toasted. To save time when using pumpkin seeds (pepitas), buy them already roasted and salted. Other nuts, such as macadamia, walnuts, almonds, and pecans should be purchased unsalted and not roasted, if possible. To toast nuts, heat an oven to 350 degrees, and bake for 8-12 minutes, until they are slightly brown and fragrant. Remember to cool the nuts completely before proceeding with your recipe.

★ *Garlic* Garlic is a very personal taste. Most people like it, but too much garlic has been known to kill a recipe. I use garlic conservatively. If you prefer a stronger garlic flavor, increase the garlic in my recipes by one clove. I also use garlic powder or McCormick Garlic and Herb Seasoning. These two spices can be used interchangeably.

Keeping Your Pantry Stocked

Here is a list of ingredients used throughout *Florida's Backyard*, that are easy to keep in your pantry or spice rack. Although you may have to purchase fresh main ingredients on the day you plan to prepare some of my recipes, with a well-stocked pantry you can whip up many of them at a moment's notice. Don't let this list intimidate you. If you are a novice and starting from scratch, merely add a few items each week and build your pantry slowly.

Spices and Herbs:
Whole Black Peppercorns
Whole White Peppercorns or Ground White Pepper
Chili Powder
Cumin
Nutmeg
Cinnamon
Cinnamon Stick
Kosher Salt
Ground Ginger
Ground Allspice
Curry Powder
California Bay Leaves
Red Pepper Flakes
Fennel Seed
Garlic Powder or McCormick Garlic and Herb Seasoning
Cayenne Pepper
Pure Vanilla Extract
Dried Oregano
Dried Thyme
Dried Rosemary
Dried Dill Weed
Dry Mustard

Non-Perishables:
Roasted Red Peppers
Green Olives
Calamata Olives

Chicken Broth (preferably low sodium)
Vegetable Broth (preferably low sodium)
Clam Juice
Canned Black Beans
Canned Kidney Beans
Chopped Tomatoes (preferably Pomi)
Marinated Artichoke Hearts
Dried Fruit, including Raisins, Golden Raisins, Cranberries, Apricots, and Figs
Sun-dried Tomatoes (preferably not in oil)
Unsweetened Coconut
Nuts, including Pecans, Walnuts, Hazelnuts (preferably skinned), and Pine Nuts
Dried, Roasted Pumpkin Seeds
Extra Virgin Olive Oil
Walnut Oil
Sesame Oil
Peanut Oil
Honey
Sugar
Brown Sugar
Pure Maple Syrup
Molasses
Vinegars, including White Wine, Red Wine, Balsamic, Raspberry, and Rice
Dijon Mustard
Honey Mustard
Hot Sauces
Strawberry or Raspberry Preserves
Mango Nectar
Seasoned Bread Crumbs
Plain Bread Crumbs
Cornstarch
Corn Meal
Chili Sauce
Capers
Soy Sauce (preferably low sodium)
Light Coconut Milk
Cooking Sherry
Dry White Cooking Wine
Hoisin Sauce
Sweetened Condensed Milk
Dutch Process Cocoa

Perishables:

These items can be purchased weekly, or on an as-needed basis. Some of these ingredients will keep in your refrigerator for up to a full week. Freezer items will keep for several months.

Frozen Corn
Frozen, Chopped Spinach
Frozen Peas
Lemons
Limes
Onions, including Vidalia, Yellow, and Red
Red and Yellow Peppers
Scallion or Green Onion
Fresh Grated Parmesan Cheese
Feta Cheese
Horseradish

Equipment Basics

Although it is fun to have kitchen gadgets, owning every culinary tool ever created is not a prerequisite to cooking a great meal. My friends and family used to get a kick out of the antique hand mixer I inherited from my grandmother. Amazingly, I created the most elaborate desserts with it. My philosophy is, "If there is a will, there is a way." However, your kitchen life *will* be easier if you keep some basic tools around.

- A good non-stick, 16-inch skillet
- Large, medium, and small saucepans
- A good stock pot with lid
- A blender or food processor
- Three basic knives: a small paring knife, an 8-to 10-inch chef's knife, and a 6-inch boning knife
- Spatula
- Whisk
- Peppermill
- Measuring spoons and cups
- Pastry brush and basting brush
- Cookie sheet
- Cheese shredder
- Grill pan or grill
- Chef's tongs
- Zester or fine grater

Fish Sense

The main reason more people don't eat fresh fish is they don't know how to select and cook it. There is no real mystery to choosing and preparing fish, so with a little bit of know-how, some tips, and practice, you can begin adding seafood to your weekly repertoire. Because there are so many varieties available today, markets are filled with fish caught locally or shipped fresh from somewhere in the U.S. Even fish from international waters make their way into most markets. So with all of this terrific fish available, it's time you learned to cook it! The first step is shopping for your catch.

Choosing the best fresh fish:

★ First, make sure your fishmonger is reputable. Ask friends and local restaurant chefs whom they recommend. Notice whether the market and its displays are clean and if the fish is well iced.

★ Ideally, you should buy the fish whole and then have it filleted. When choosing a fish, check its eyes, which should be clear. If there is film on the eyes, the fish will be less than fresh.

★ Fish should *not* have a strong odor. It should smell like fish, but the odor should not be offensive.

★ If you are buying fish already filleted, ask when it was caught. Ask if you can smell the filet or if you can touch it through a plastic covering. The filet should be firm, not mushy. If the filet shows any signs of foaming, like soap, it is old and should not be eaten.

★ Always keep your fish well-iced. If you aren't going straight home after you leave the market, take a cooler with you and ask your fishmonger to pack your fish in ice for the road.

Available fish and easy substitutions:

★ **Dolphin (Mahi-Mahi)** We Floridians have always called this fish a Dolphin, with the understanding that it bears no resemblance to "Flipper," the celebrity mammal. However, to avoid confusion among tourists and newcomers, this firm, large-flaked fish has been given the moniker "mahi-mahi." Dolphinfish is a beautiful color, with brilliant blue-green skin that turns silver and yellow after the fish is caught. *Good substitutions: Monkfish, Atlantic Halibut, and Sole.*

★ **Grouper** This firm, white-fleshed fish is a favorite of seafood lovers. It has a mild flavor, and can be grilled, sautéed, baked, broiled or even stir-fried, with excellent results. There are numerous members of the grouper family, but the tastiest include Strawberry Grouper, Gray Grouper, Yellowfin Grouper, and Red Grouper. With the exception of the Strawberry Grouper, they can all grow to be quite large, but smaller fish have a sweeter flavor. *Good substitutions: Sea Bass, Cobia or Hogfish.*

★ **Native (Florida) Snapper** Nothing compares to the sweet, flaky taste of the Native (Florida) Snapper. Plus, snappers are as much fun to catch as they are to eat. The best and most popular varieties include Yellowtail Snapper, Mutton Snapper (called Red Snapper because it turns a brilliant reddish-pink after it's caught), Mangrove Snapper, Gray Snapper,

Trippletail, and Hogfish (not a true snapper, although it's commonly referred to as Hog Snapper). *Good substitutions: Tilapia, Sole, Striped Bass, and Rockfish.*

★ **Tuna** Tuna has gained heavily in popularity, due to its lean meat, dense flavor, and importance to ever-popular Asian cuisine. We often catch Yellowfin Tuna, which is among the tastiest of the Tuna varieties, in the Bahamas and off the Florida coast. *Good substitutions: Because Tuna has a distinctive flavor, any substitutions you make will alter the integrity of your recipe. But other "steak" variety fish you can use include Wahoo and Swordfish.*

★ **Cobia** This is one of my Florida favorites, and it's definitely in a class by itself! Firm, white and mildly flavored, Cobia adapts to the grill easily and is usually cut steak-style. It cooks well in a wok because it holds together in solid pieces. *Good substitutions: Grouper, Swordfish, Mahi-Mahi, and Hogfish.*

★ **Shrimp and Shellfish** A good variety of shrimp and scallops is available throughout the world. Shrimp are usually pre-frozen, which should not impact their flavor because they freeze well. Remember when buying shrimp and scallops that they should not have a strong odor or feel slimy.

★ **Florida Lobster** This delicious crustacean is widely available throughout the Southeast. It is native to the warm waters of Florida and the Caribbean, where it's caught from August until January. If you are buying shellfish during the off-season, it will have been pre-frozen. *Good substitutions: Maine lobster or rock shrimp.*

★ **Conch** (pronounced konk) This is one tough crustacean! Conch, which is frequently available in good fish markets, is a white, sweet shellfish native to the warm waters of Florida and the Caribbean. Conch are endangered in Florida, where sportsmen are prohibited from diving for them. So unless you are diving for fresh conch off the Bahamas, your conch will most likely be frozen, which will not impact its flavor. To prepare it, place it in a plastic baggy and pound it with a mallet to about ¼-inch thickness. It's okay if the meat starts to fall apart. *Good substitutions: It's difficult to identify a true substitute for conch, because its flavor and texture are so distinct. In a pinch, however, clams or bay scallops will work in some recipes that call for conch.*

Slimming Down Your Recipes

If you are on a low-fat or low-sodium diet, you can adapt many of my recipes by using low-fat or reduced-fat ingredients. In general, my recipes use very little fat, because I rely on fresh herbs, fruits, fruit juices and the best ingredients to create flavorful dishes. However, here are some basic substitutions you can make to reduce fat, cut calories or reduce sodium:

★ Use reduced-fat sour cream instead of regular sour cream.
★ Use light or reduced-fat butter instead of butter when sautéing. Or use 1 teaspoon of olive oil or olive oil cooking spray for sautéing. Do *not* use reduced fat butter when baking. My preferred brand of light butter is Land of Lakes.
★ Use reduced-fat or low-fat mayonnaise instead of regular mayonnaise.
★ Substitute skim milk for whole or reduced-fat milk.
★ Interchange plain yogurt and low-fat buttermilk.
★ Sauté in a non-stick skillet so you can cut the required amount of butter or oil in half.
★ Use half the amount of nuts or seeds in any recipe.
★ Use salt sparingly and season recipes only to taste.
★ Use low-sodium soy sauce instead of regular soy sauce

Chapter 7:

Foolproof Entertaining

I have always been known as a "party girl." By that, I mean I find parties magical and love everything about them, whether I'm hosting, helping friends or attending. Hosting parties is second nature to me, but I realize this is not the case for everyone. So, this chapter is for those of you who want to learn how to host *and* enjoy a great party.

Here are the key elements to throwing a terrific party: a well-thought-out guest list, good food, the right music, and a welcoming atmosphere. Last, but not least: Be a relaxed host. By that I mean don't make the mistake of being too busy with the details to enjoy your own party, causing the atmosphere and spirit of the party to suffer. The lesson here is simple. A harried host makes for a less-than-comfortable setting. Fortunately, however, with proper planning and my foolproof checklist, you *can* host a perfect event!

Party Checklist

★ **The Guest List** This is the cornerstone of your event, so think hard about whom you are inviting and the purpose behind the party. For example, do you want to give a party to introduce new people to each other? If so, do they have common interests? Will they like each other? How will you get the conversation going? What conversational tools can you use to prompt discussion (travel, art, theater, movies, food)?

Try to bring together an interesting mix of people. Think about the personalities of your guests and who will match well with whom. Make sure you have a good mix of extroverts in your group to help draw out any introverts. If you're planning a seated meal, mix up the couples; it's the best way to introduce new topics of discussion and prevent the evening from becoming a competitive discussion about children. Not that I am against talking about kids, but this subject can consume an entire evening and will eventually bore some people.

If the party is for business, think about how you can group people so they don't just talk shop all evening; successful business parties do not drown in office talk. The key is to build relationships through the evening and save the hard-core business matters for the office. Finally, remember that your role will be to make sure that people meet each other, that you identify their common interests, and that you talk to everyone at some point during the evening, even if it's for five minutes.

★ **Invitations** The importance of the party invitation is often overlooked. A party invitation should entice and interest your guests, while making them feel special for being invited. This does not, however, mean you must send an engraved invitation. Actually, the invitation should reflect your own personality, as well as the theme and character of the event. The size of the party will also dictate the method by which you will invite your guests.

For example, a dinner party for 14 or fewer people does not require a written invitation. A telephone invitation for a dinner party of this size is acceptable, and should be made two weeks prior to the event. Any party over ten couples or 20 people requires a written invitation. The only exception is a party honoring someone, such as a bridal shower, baby shower or an engagement party. In these cases, regardless of the number of guests, a written invitation is a must.

Be creative with your printed or written invitations, especially for a casual party or themed event. Creative invitations will set the tone for a fun event and establish the character of your party. If you are having a more formal event, keep your invitations simple, and choose beautiful paper, a classic ink color, and a simple pattern. In our high-tech world of convenience, e-mail invitations are becoming increasingly popular. However, use of this contemporary time-saver should be kept to a minimum and reserved for extremely casual gatherings. Nothing can replace the warm touch of a personal phone call, a hand-written invitation or a creatively printed piece.

★ **RSVP** It is an absolute requirement to include an RSVP on any printed invitation. Using "Regrets Only" or accepting all responses is an individual preference. But in order to eliminate confusion, I require every invitee to respond. Track your RSVPs by keeping a printout of your invitation list by your phone. Then, whoever answers the phone can easily make a notation on the list. E-mail is an acceptable form of response, but keep in mind that if you include your e-mail address, you should check your e-messages frequently.

If you invite 75 persons or more, it is a fact that some people will not respond to your invitation. Also, some people who said they would attend, won't, and some people who said they would not attend, will. This is just the way of the world. To be prepared for this scenario, calculate your numbers for seating or food, by assuming that 10 percent of your invitees will not show. If you received a response from all your guests, adjust your numbers accordingly. If you did not receive a response from all your guests, then you have two ways to calculate attendance: (1) Assume that 10% of those who did not respond will show up, and keep your count the same, or (2) Call those who did not respond and ask them if they are coming. Either method will give you an accurate count.

★ **Entertainment** This is the trickiest part of setting the tone for the evening. It's not always necessary to have live music or expensive entertainment to have a successful party. But it *is* necessary to be creative. Music is the most essential ingredient, unless you are gathering to watch a sporting event. So select your music in advance and make sure your sound system is in good working order. If you are serving a meal, select mood-setting music rather than rock and roll. If you hire musicians, tell them in advance exactly what you want played. Or give them a song list or description of the party so they'll know what's appropriate to play and when. Tell your musicians during a break to change their format, if they don't set the mood you want. And if you want people to dance, make sure to designate a specific, convenient area, where they'll feel comfortable.

Finally, if you don't have music, find other activities to keep your party lively and active. For example, add a card game, a trivial pursuit game or even conversational games. Remember, your guests are there to relax and get away from everyday pressures, so it's up to you to provide the proper distractions.

★ **Table Settings and Decorations** The atmosphere and setting you create at your party can be simple or elaborate, but most importantly, it should reflect your personal style. I am not one to go to extremes with decorations, preferring to rely on natural settings, beautiful flower arrangements, strategically placed candles, and colorful tablecloths. There are many options for creating a setting that fits your party theme. The basics are as follows:

- Flower arrangements and candles
- Tablecloths and napkins
- Tableware and glasses
- Bar settings and equipment, including champagne buckets, ice buckets or a wine bucket
- Lighting, outdoors and indoors

If you choose to embellish, keep it simple. If your home is properly decorated, there is no need to add elements that could detract from its décor.

Instead, think of ways in which your tableware can add character. For a casual party, indoors or out, select colorful plates and napkins and less formal tableware. If you are hosting a formal event, use white linens, formal china and your best crystal.

★ **Food and Beverages** Now it's time to get serious. You have your guest list, invitations, and music. What on earth are you going to serve? Analyze your menu as it relates to your guests and their preferences. For a small dinner gathering, have a sense of what your guests like and consider any food allergies your guests might have. If you're having a large dinner or cocktail party, offer enough variety to satisfy more than one type of taste, remembering to include vegetarians, as well as beef and seafood lovers.

Beverages should also accommodate the likes and dislikes of your guests. If you are having guests who don't drink wine, it's best to offer a full bar, large or small, set up to include the following spirits:

Minimum Bar
Gin
Vodka
Dark Rum (real rum drinkers prefer a dark rum such as Mount Gay, Anejo Supreme or Captain Morgan)
Scotch
Bourbon or Whiskey
Red Wine
White Wine such as a Chardonnay or Pinot Grigio
Beer (both regular and light)

Mixers should include the following:
Tonic
Coke and Diet Coke
Cranberry Juice
Sparkling Water
Grapefruit or Orange Juice
Limes and Lemons

Expanded Bar
Include all of the liquor listed above and add the following spirits and mixers:
Kahlua
Extra Dry Vermouth (for martinis)
Triple Sec
Tequila
Sour Mix
Ginger Ale
Apricot or Flavored Brandy

Pineapple Juice
Milk
Orange Slices
Olives
Tomolives

If your guests like wine, offer a variety of wines and beers and eliminate the liquor. Champagne adds a festive touch, but is not necessary, unless the celebration is a wedding or an anniversary. Of course, champagne is always appropriate at any holiday event.

★ **The Menu** My absolute favorite part of planning a party is creating the menu. I typically pick a menu to match the theme of the event, such as Asian, Latin, Backyard Barbecue, Caribbean, Seafood Fest, and so forth, then carry it through all the details. When simplicity is in order, however, a great pasta meal with salad, bread, and dessert can be just right, too. Here are several menus to give you some ideas about how to combine the recipes in *Florida's Backyard* to create a fun and memorable party. Remember, you don't have to make every dish yourself. Outsourcing part of the menu is the right thing to do if you are pressed for time.

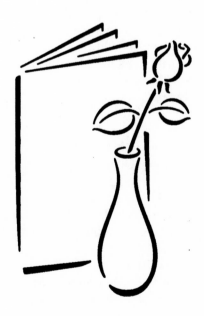

Party Menus from *Florida's Backyard*

Here, I have chosen several occasions and suggested a menu for each:

Boat Cruise Light Dinner
Lobster Cocktail with Mustard Sauce
Avocado Bruschetta
Asparagus and Tomato Salad
Summer Primavera Salad
Cornmeal-Crusted Shrimp with Jalapeño Jelly
Cookies and Brownies (purchased)

Bahamas Bash
Abaco Conch Fritters with Two Sauces
Beer-Battered Bahamian Crawfish
Wild Greens with Mango Vinaigrette
Crispy Yellowtail Parmesan
Island Rice
Beehive Coconut Pie

Caribbean Dinner Party for 12
Endive Spears with Goat Cheese and Pineapple
Asparagus with Dilled Yogurt Horseradish Dip
Chilled Roasted Pepper and Mango Soup
Summer Salad with Lemon Basil Ginger Vinaigrette
Grilled Cobia with Papaya Salsa
Sun-kissed Couscous
Tropical Fruit Pizza

Casual Back Deck Cocktails for 20
Triple Cheese Shrimp Quesadilla
Avocado Bruschetta
Cornmeal-Crusted Shrimp with Jalapeno Jelly
Endive Spears with Goat Cheese and Pineapple
Red Wine Infused Beef Kabobs (in miniature)

Nuevo Latino Dinner for 12
Selection of Spanish Olives (purchased)
Manchego Cheese Tray with Crisp Crackers (purchased)
Avocado and Roasted Corn Soup

Pan-Seared Scallops with Papaya-Yellow Tomato Salsa (appetizer portions)
Grilled Mambo Chicken with Red Pepper Coulis
Crispy Jalapeno Olive Potatoes
Flan de La Finca

Family Backyard Barbeque for 12
Spinach Salad with Warm Strawberry Vinaigrette
Mango Barbeque Chicken
Bourbon and Balsamic Barbeque Pork Tenderloin
Soulful Succotash
Corn Bread (purchased)
Frozen Lime Pie

Tropical Sunday Brunch
Bread Basket, including Lavosh, Mini-fruit Muffins, Whole Grain and French Rolls (purchased)
Carrot Ginger Soup
Mixed Greens and Berries with Honey-Laced Citrus Vinaigrette
Grilled Chicken Pasta Salad with Light Peanut Dressing
Skinny Crab and Asparagus Quiche
Banana Coconut Rum Cake

Florida Holiday Menu
Avocado Bruschetta
Smoky Sweet Potato Soup
Spinach and Dried Fruit Salad with Lemon Vinaigrette
Pan-Seared Colossal Shrimp with Cranberry-Orange Salsa
Nutty Island Rice
Creamsicle Chiffon Pie

Remember, the secret to having fun at your own party is planning ahead. Following the party guidelines and using the delicious, easy-to-fix recipes in *Florida's Backyard* will make the preparations really easy, *and* put you on track to hosting a successful party. So all you have to do is enjoy!

Bibliography

Caroline Stuart and Jeanne Voltz, Florida Cookbook: From Gulf Coast Gumbo to Key Lime Pie. Alfred A. Knopf, New York, NY, 1993.

Rae Shelley Drew, Cooking with Florida Citrus. Drummond Press, NY, 1998.

Jerry Traunfeld, The Herbfarm Cookbook. Scribner, New York, NY, 2000.

Allen Susser, New World Cuisine, Doubleday, New York, NY, 1995.

Recipe Index

Printed in the United States
38572LVS00005B/202-324

9 780759 648029